A Guide to a Pain,

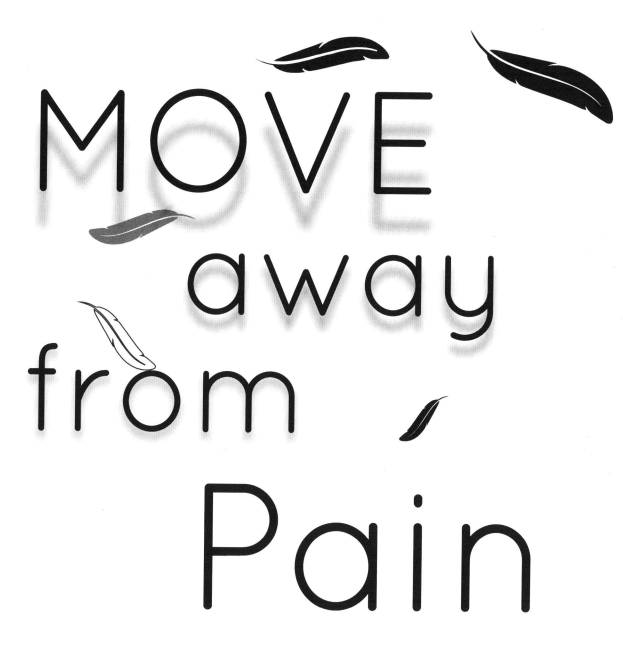

MOVE away from Pain

Marie-Claire Prettyman

MOVE Away From Pain

First published in 2020 by

Panoma Press Ltd
48 St Vincent Drive, St Albans, Herts, AL1 5SJ, UK
info@panomapress.com
www.panomapress.com

Book layout by Neil Coe.

978-1-784529-05-5

A CIP catalogue record for this book is available from the British Library.

This book is available online and in bookstores.

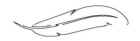

Acknowledgments

Thank you!

Huge thanks as always to the creative people in my life:

Katey Fox for your brilliant photography as always
www.kateyfoxphotography.co.uk

Clare Green for such cute illustrations
www.fromlenstocanvas.co.uk

and to

Susannah Thompson for helping me write in less jargon and
stopping my grammatical tick! (Parenthesis)

Finally, thanks to my husband and son for making me tea and
putting up with me when I shut myself away for days on end
because I've had a 'good idea'.

I love you loads xx

Contents

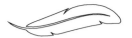

The Personal Bit

After I hurt/broke some bits of my back and pelvis falling on to a tiled floor in a leisure centre I fully expected to be completely fine within a couple of days; but then it was weeks, then months and the pain didn't get better, it got worse.

I owned a Pilates and Yoga studio, I ran Pilates and Yoga teacher training courses, I was (still am) a mum and really needed to be the strongest and most powerful version of myself to do it all, but I just couldn't.

The pain kept me up at night, I worried about it, wondering what on earth I had done to myself to be suffering so badly. I became depressed and lost confidence in my abilities to do my job; eventually this all culminated in me having to sell my business and do something else for a while. I went to work in a school as a teaching assistant, but I was so depleted in energy and confidence I couldn't even do that after a while. I suffered from anxiety, depression and fatigue.

I did, however, find some excellent pain management medics, who through a number of nerve ablations and steroid injections prevented a proposed surgery and allowed me to get off all the pain medication, including morphine. The reduction of pain allowed me to start moving properly again, and as a result I got stronger and stronger and I moved away from *my* pain.

All of this sparked an interest in working with others who were suffering from chronic pain, so I started to do more reading and attend courses on pain management and therapeutic interventions for pain, and it was here that I actually started to learn what I feel I should have known four years previously.

I had understood that the pain medication was there to help me move more freely so that my body could heal, but the deep impact of stress and worry on my pain receptors was not fully explained (or if it was, I hadn't been able to process it). The way that pain behaves as a separate entity to injury was not clear. Retraining PAIN as opposed to fixing musculoskeletal damage was not clear (at the time).

It felt at times that people around me thought it was all in my head (it was) but not in a psychological 'made it all up' kind of way, but the pain *was* being created by the brain, certainly. I know that if you're reading this, then you've experienced a similar issue. You've felt 'not listened to' or dismissed; that somehow people aren't believing you with respect to how much you are suffering.

I want this book to explain the things I've learned over the last couple of years so that someone else doesn't have to spend years fighting the system and themselves in order to move forward. Learning about pain can help you manage it and MOVE past it.

The exercises are a combination of Pilates and Yoga inspired actions, designed to gently encourage your body to let go of its excitable pain signals and relax into comfortable pain-free movements. MOVING is the key so that:

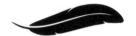

YOU can control your pain

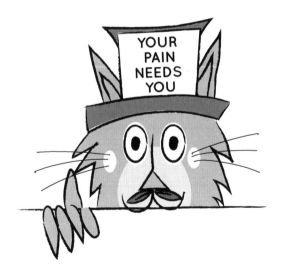

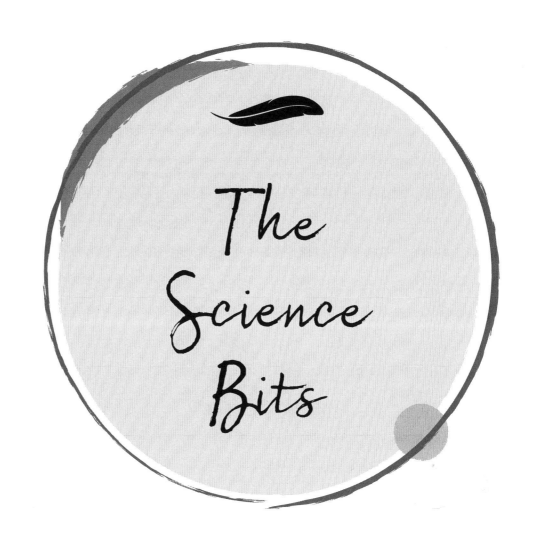

The
Science
Bits

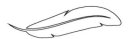

Science Bit 1

Pain is Weird

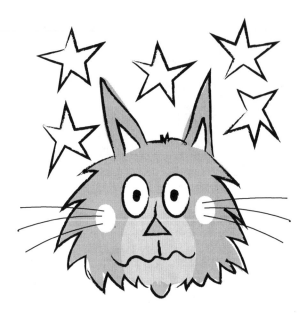

Long-term pain isn't just about what is going on in your body, despite what it might feel like. There are many other factors involved as you'll see working your way through this book.

I remember being told years ago that 'pain is your body's warning system, it's telling you to stop doing what you are doing'; well, sometimes this is true, sometimes it's not!

Many people still believe that ceasing activity is an appropriate management strategy for pain, for fear of further harming oneself. There are very rare cases where this might be true, but most often, rest and avoidance practices are the exact opposite of what is needed.

Dr Eyal Lederman divides recovery from pain/injury into three overlapping sections: repair, adaptation and alleviation of symptoms with 'recovery' in the middle.

For example, if a person sprains their ankle, their recovery would be expected to take place through a process of tissue repair (repair – usually six to eight weeks); pain during this phase is definitely a message to cease or moderate activities until it's feeling better.

If the ankle was immobilised following an ankle fracture, multisystem adaptive changes would need to take place rather than just repairing tissues (adaptation).

The most interesting section in the management of long-term, chronic pain conditions however is the last one. Take a person who experiences chronic back pain for several months and within a few weeks of an intervention treatment like osteopathy/chiropractic/physiotherapy or sports massage the person experiences a dramatic improvement in symptoms.

If that individual had an MRI at the start of treatment and another at the end, the findings would very likely remain unchanged. As Dr Lederman states, "It can therefore be assumed that their recovery is related to reduction of the amplitude of their symptoms rather than by tissue repair or adaptation."

As mentioned, these three processes do overlap, particularly between 'repair' and 'alleviation of symptoms' during the recovery from acute conditions e.g. following an ankle sprain.

- The ankle gets better due to the tissues healing and a subsequent reduction in symptoms.

The recovery from chronic conditions like lower back pain however is represented by the overlap between 'alleviation of symptoms' and 'adaptation'.

- The back gets better due to a combination of complicated neurological, lymphatic and muscular adaptations within the body whilst simultaneously calming the symptoms.

Chronic pain is associated with ***central nervous system sensitivity***, to deal with it; recovery interventions need to include a long-term commitment to desensitising the nervous system through calming activities (see the section on Relaxation Techniques), treatments, movement protocols and support.

This concept moves us a long way away from the biomechanical/ structural model of assuming that there is a 'correct' position for our bodies to be in, in order to reduce pain and facilitate function.

Countless studies have found little evidence between pain and pathologies, so we can deduce:

PAIN is not just about DAMAGE

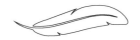

Science Bit 2

Nociception

'The central nervous system's response to certain harmful or potentially harmful stimuli.'

All round our bodies we have sensors that give us lots of information. Like most information, some of it is useful, but we have to make a decision about what any particular piece of information means.

Nociceptors (sensory receptors) in particular respond to physical, chemical or temperature stressors. Sometimes nociception leads to pain. If you put your hand near a fire, your temperature nociceptors might signal that the hand is too hot and that you need to move it or you'll burn yourself. You may experience some pain, you will probably move the hand, but you don't have any damage here.

Nociception is well related to pain and damage immediately following an injury. Like during the 'repair' phase of the process approach, the signals are there to ensure you rest and do not aggravate the injury. But after a while, the relationship between healthy nociception as a warning signal and pain becomes less strong. You can start to have more pain, with less nociception (stimulations of the receptors), or pain with the same amount of nociception, or even pain with no nociception at all!

So herein lies the problem with nociception. When they send their potential warning signals to the spinal cord, the spinal cord can act like an amplifier where it can turn the signal up and send the message to the brain. Or it can be turned down, and less signal gets sent to the brain.

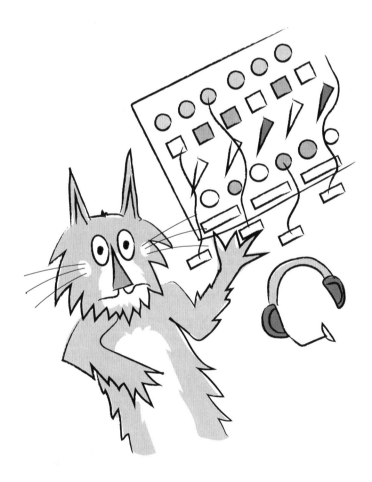

If the spinal cord gets confused (like a switchboard operator) it may start sending signals that are simply about touch or pressure, as nociception and now the brain thinks that something less important is potentially dangerous. Now instead of just a gentle sensation, the message reads 'PAIN'.

Pain is so much more than just nociception; it's just a potential warning signal. Your brain has to make decisions about what to do with that warning signal, and it's affected by expectations, beliefs, past experiences and attitude.

Other issues associated with the pain-giving event, like muscle tightness and stress, can contribute to the amount of pain felt at any one moment, even if the level of nociception is the same or even less than at another potentially injuring time/event.

The greater the stress on the brain at the time, the greater potential there is for an amplified pain signal.

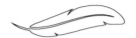

Science Bit 3

Habit

So, as we've seen, pain can be affected by other triggers like stress (physical and/or psychological), and as pain persists, it becomes more about the triggers of sensitivity and less about any damage or nociception from the tissues. In effect, the pain has become like a habit.

You start to create links in your brain pertaining to certain activities and pain, e.g. sitting on a chair for too long, or going for too long a walk. These links become detrimental and enforce avoidance behaviours.

Associating any type of movement or activity with pain will drive a certain amount of fear or worry and so it's important to break that association carefully, maybe by doing things more slowly or differently. Gradually, you can create new, more positive associations with these movements or activities and enjoy them without sensitivity related pain.

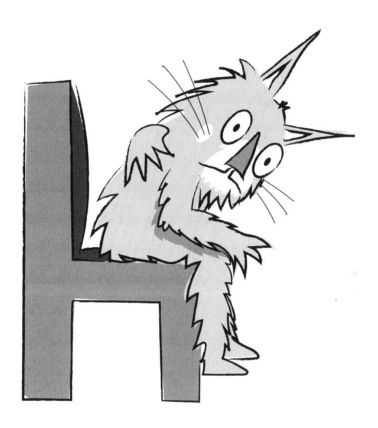

Pain is a HABIT we need to break

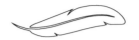

Science Bit 4

Sensitivity

People with 'centralised' sensitivity will often find that pain moves around the body, and they may also be sensitive to light or foods. They will also feel pain where they should really only feel pressure or touch. These people also tend to suffer 'flare-ups' more readily.

Some people who have 'milder' or 'intermittent' pain can feel better through exercise or activities like foam rolling, thanks to the activation of a process which exerts a modifying or controlling influence on nociception, and creates an internally generated analgesia (pain relief).

Those with 'centralised' sensitisation often have no positive response to these approaches and if they try, can experience flare-ups with even more pain. They lose the ability to control the irritation. However, exercise is still important, we just have to do it differently, slowly progress the intensity over a long period of time and accept that:

Some flare-ups and discomfort will occur

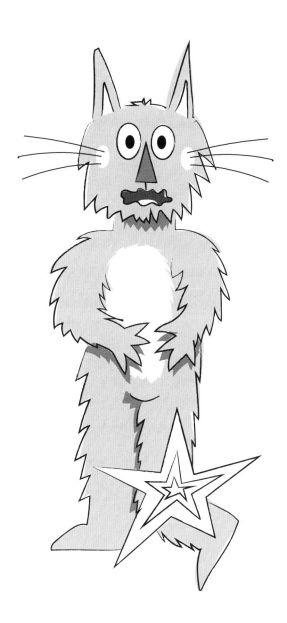

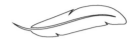

Science Bit 5

Perception

It's very unlikely (unless you have dislocated your shoulder or something similar) that you have a joint out of place. But it is common to feel that something just 'isn't right'. The brain controls movement and your perception of your body, but with persistent pain your recognition of where all your body parts are and how they are functioning becomes distorted.

You may start to feel like your joints are 'out of place' or you feel weakness in random areas; this can all be retrained to work more symbiotically over time.

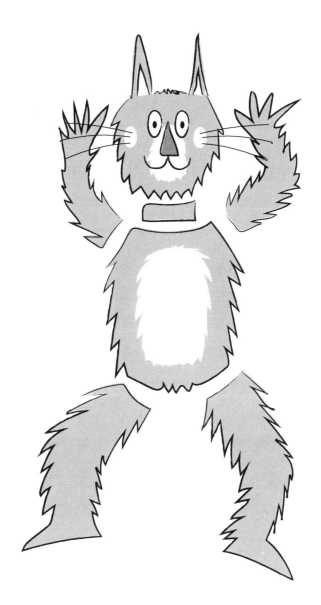

You are not OUT OF PLACE

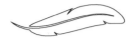

Science Bit 6

Adaptability

Our spines are amazing, they can withstand more than 2000lbs of pressure! Most of the activities we undertake in our daily lives are far below the maximal threshold where tissue gets injured, yet more people who have pain will have been told that they are weak or tight, or that something is 'unstable'.

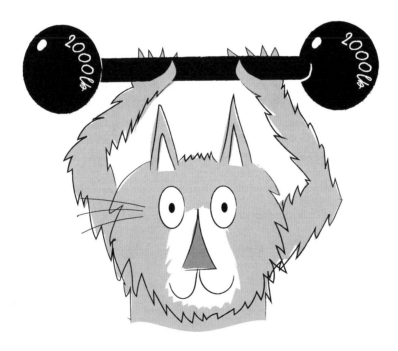

Pain is poorly explained by your strength. Humans are adaptable: you adapted to get into pain and you will adapt to get out of it. The longer you adapted *into* your pain, the longer it will take you to adapt out of it.

Exercise or any activity that makes you stronger is great for managing pain, but not usually for the reasons people think i.e. gaining muscular strength.

Just changing the perception you have of your body from one that is 'weak' and/or 'ineffective' to being capable and strong can, on its own, help with pain. It is important to build up tolerance to irritating activities to develop a resilience to sensitivity. Have patience though:

It's a marathon not a sprint

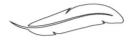

Science Bit 7

Flexibility

Flexibility is poorly related to pain in the same way that so-called 'muscle weakness' is not related to pain.

If your lower back hurts when you bend forwards, you could avoid that action for a while to see if the sensitivity 'calms down'. If the hamstrings are so tight that a person cannot avoid bending forwards when moving, the lower back may continue to be irritated. In this way potentially, poor flexibility could be an aggravating factor, but in general most people who are tight have no pain. People who are loose have no pain and equally both these groups can have pain.

However, undertaking strengthening and stretching activities are excellent ways to improve sensitivity at the end of a joint range of motion and can therefore have an effect on centralised sensitivity, subsequently reducing pain overall. Just remember though:

It's not your inability to touch your toes
that's causing your pain...

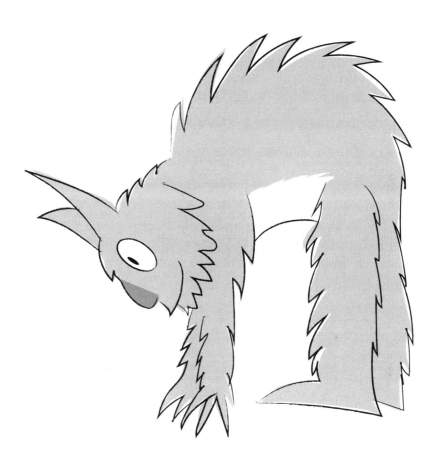

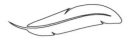

Science Bit 8

Posture

Your 'posture' is not causing your pain either (despite what you may have been told!). Sitting for long periods of time in the same position can cause discomfort, sure, but when you get up and move around it eases. There isn't a perfect sitting position to prevent this from happening, you just need to respond to the message you are being sent and reduce the momentary irritation.

- Most people have one shoulder lower than the other, they don't have pain.

- Many people have a scoliosis, they don't have pain.

- Many people have a minor leg length discrepancy, they don't have pain.

- Lots of people have 'rounded shoulders', they don't have pain.

Our bodies are biological not mechanical and we can adapt, adapt, adapt!

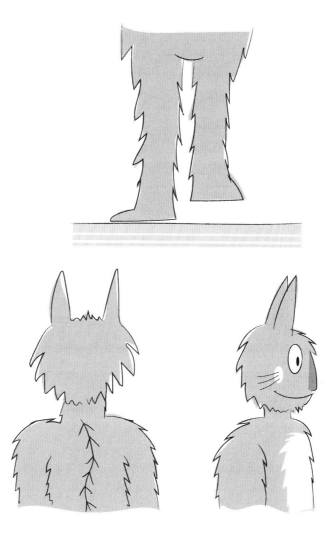

Try not to fixate on so-called 'correct' ways of sitting/standing/walking, just move around a bit if you're uncomfortable. Move desks for half an hour, stand up and type – it doesn't matter. But engaging with the doctrine of 'sitting is bad for your back and that's why I have a bad back' is amplifying the sensitivity through beliefs!

Your posture is NOT causing your pain

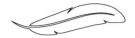

Science Bit 9

Stress

Pain is often associated with a stressful event, and as a result later episodes of stress and the associated chemical release can trigger the same pain (as seen in the 'Habit' section). I have heard so many times a client telling me all about their problems at work, with a partner and/or kids etc. and then following up with "...and now my sciatica's flared up again!" It's not that there's another injury, or even an exacerbation of an old injury, it's simply the related chemicals triggering a previous pain link to stress.

We cannot avoid stress or stressors, it's a normal part of life. We can help manage this though through regular practice of relaxation (see Relaxation Techniques section).

It is also normal to have random pains, like sharp stabbing pains in the knee or a similar pain in the back; these are normal, it doesn't mean you've harmed yourself. The worst thing you can do in that situation is start fretting about what it might mean...

Kids
Family
Work
Weight
Health
Money

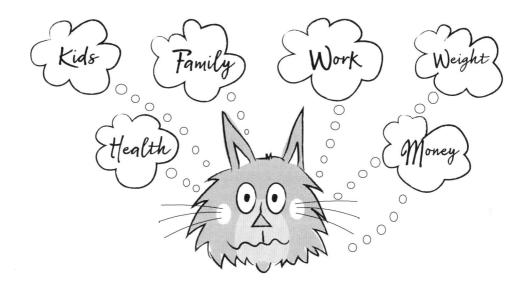

...let it go, the pain is transient...

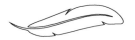

Science Bit 10

Degeneration

One of my favourite quotes is *'Degeneration is like having wrinkles on the inside'* – Dr Greg Lehman.

Many people have scans of their painful joints which show up things like bone spurs or microtears on to which we can hang all of our pain and discomfort and feel totally validated. But guess what?

Everyone has these things and for the most part they are totally *irrelevant*. They are not 'abnormalities', they are 'normalities' and are very poorly related to pain.

One particular study asked surgeons to scan the so-called 'healthy joint' in opposition to any joint that they may or may not be going to operate on to see what the difference was. In many cases the joint without pain showed similar levels, if not more, of so-called 'degeneration' or damage, implying that the identified 'damage' was not in fact causing the pain at all!

In a few TV documentaries over the years, surgeons involved in various randomised trials exploring the 'placebo effect' were asked either to go ahead with a proposed surgery or not, depending on into which group the patient was allocated.

Two patients who did not have their surgery spring to mind. The first thought she'd had bone spurs removed from her shoulder. She was interviewed using a hedge trimmer months later, commenting that she couldn't have done any of what she was doing before her operation *(she did not have the operation, she just thought she had).*

Another was a lady in the USA who thought she'd had a type of cement injected into her vertebra following a fracture that left her in severe pain; she could be seen two weeks later playing golf, pain free. *She did not have the procedure, she just thought she'd had the procedure!*

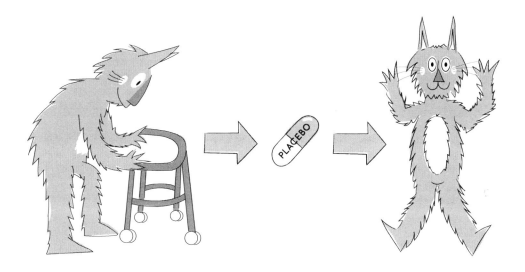

My point is this: being told you 'have something' isn't always the most useful piece of information; it can cause further sensitivity thanks to those belief systems and protective/avoidance behaviours.

These two ladies had a more positive attitude because they thought that someone had 'fixed them'. * see next section

So, a positive attitude to reducing sensitivity and not fixating on 'damage' is how you move forward.

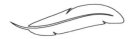

Science Bit Finale

You don't need fixing

I'm not saying a bit of support from a manual therapist isn't helpful – for many people it is, but they are not 'fixing you'. They are supporting you in your self-efficacy, your belief that you can succeed in managing your situation. Touch is extremely powerful and calming to the central nervous system and so it has great value in 'alleviating symptoms' (remember Dr Lederman's process approach?).

With a reduction in pain you can explore movement more freely and work on reducing your sensitive reactions to triggers. Manual therapists will be there for you as long as you need them and for those random times over the years when you need to revisit. But ultimately managing your pain is your journey and it starts here, with establishing movement patterns and learning to enjoy your body once again.

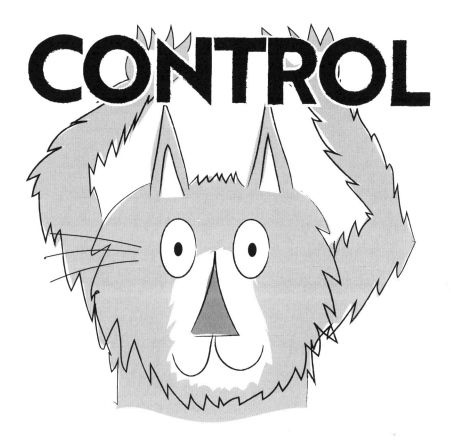

CONTROL

You've got this!

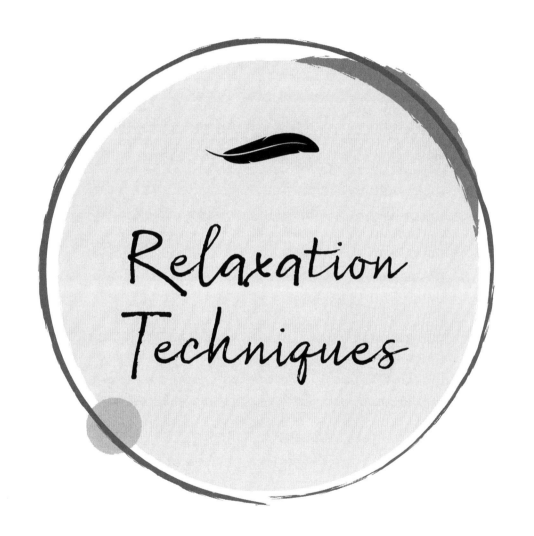

Relaxation Techniques

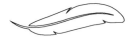

Relaxation Techniques

According to George A. Miller (1956) in his short-term memory research, we are capable of retaining seven pieces of information (plus or minus two).

Pain is notorious for affecting our ability to function at optimum levels, and for that reason these practices will only require you to remember five *simple* instructions so that you can just settle into your relaxation experience without having to repeatedly check the details.

It is more common to practise relaxation at the **end** of a movement activity, however in this instance I am asking that you practise relaxation first, to calm the central nervous system and settle your pain sensors in order to get the most out of your exercises.

As you get to know the relaxation techniques and improve, you can increase the amount of time you practise and experience a greater sense of peace as a result. Hopefully this will lead to a more positive outlook with regards to movement, both with these exercises and with life in general.

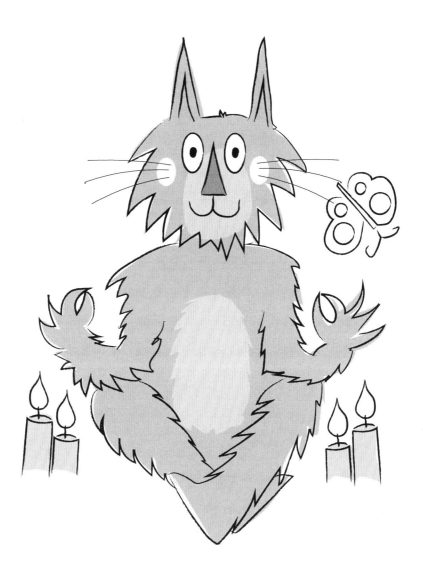

TO START

Choose a very gentle alarm, perhaps using your phone. It isn't pleasant to be hauled out of relaxation by an aggressive sound. Personally, I like the sounds of the rainforest or the sea; choose something that makes you smile or something that generates a positive old memory.

Choose a technique to practise and read the directions a few times before settling down into a comfortable position, lying down or sitting, whatever feels best to you.

Make sure that you will not be interrupted

Start with five minutes, build up to seven and then 10. Anything longer than 10 minutes might make you too groggy for your practice. However, you could practise again after your exercises for as long as you like and also independently of the exercises.

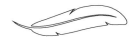

Relaxation 1:
The Breath

Learn this one first, before attempting the others.

From YOUR comfortable position:

- Bring your attention to deepening and smoothing out the breath.

- Observe the path of the breath as it travels IN through the nose, down through the lungs and then into the belly. Allow the belly to softly rise.

- Observe the path of the breath as it travels OUT of the body, from the belly, through the lungs and then out through the nose.

- Keep your attention on the breath, but allow your whole body to soften and release as the breath slows and deepens.

- If your mind starts to drift away from the breath and the sense of release in your body, acknowledge the thought without judgment, and then gently bring the attention back to the task of relaxation.

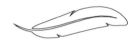

Relaxation 2:
Awareness of the Physical Body

From YOUR comfortable position:

- After relaxing the breath, bring your attention to a sense of heaviness and warmth in your right hand and right arm. Notice everything about your right hand and arm. Notice how calm it feels.

- Now do the same with the left hand and arm.

- Bring your attention now to your right foot and leg.

- And now your left foot and leg.

- Allow your whole body to feel heavy, warm and calm.

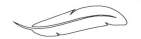

Relaxation 3:
The Meadow

From YOUR comfortable position:

- After relaxing the breath, imagine yourself sitting or lying in a meadow in gentle warming sunshine.

- Feel the soft, velvety, freshly mown grass.

- Hear the gentle chirp of the birds in the trees.

- You are completely safe and alone in this space.

- As the sun shines softly on your face, give yourself permission to let go. Become the observer of your own relaxation.

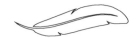

Relaxation 4:

The Beach

From LYING DOWN:

- After relaxing the breath, imagine yourself lying on soft, warming sand.

- Your body sinks gently into the sand as the sun shines gently on to your face.

- Listen to the gentle sounds of the sea lapping against the shore.

- Are there other sounds? Do you hear children laughing? Seagulls?

- Your breath is calm, your body is heavy, you are at peace in this space.

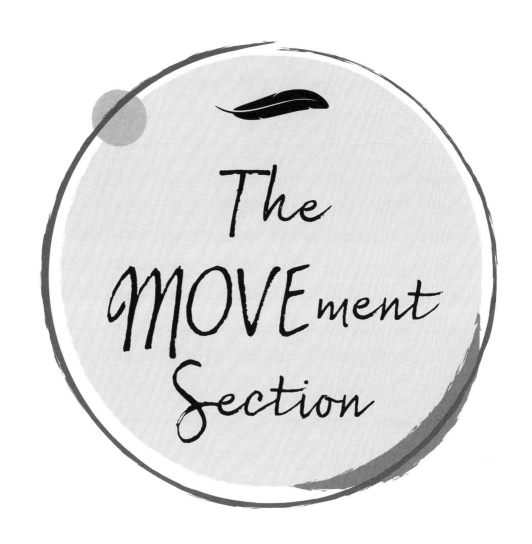

The
MOVEment
Section

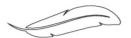

With regards to your pain, go to it, not through it...

Challenge yourself a little, but not so much that your pain signals are amplified for potentially hours or days afterwards.

Work *with* your breath, my Yoga teacher once told me:

> **'Whilst you still have your breath, nobody can steal your peace'** which I believe matters here, as we are looking for neurological peace in order to create physical peace.

The calming of your breath will settle an excitable nervous system, and so has enormous value in managing/reducing pain.

Each body part is divided into *three* sections of **five** exercises:

'The Beginning', 'Improving' and *'Getting Better'*

Choose from **'The Back', 'The Hips', 'The Shoulders', 'The Knees', 'The Elbows', 'The Ankles and Feet'** and **'The Wrists and Hands'.**

You only need to move on when you are ready and you can repeat these exercises as often as you like.

Once you have completed 'Getting Better' for your particular body section of interest, you can combine routines to create more of a whole-body workout, rather than a rehabilitation practice.

e.g. Start with *'The Beginning'* of **'The Hands and Feet'**

Continue with *'Improving for'* **'The Shoulders'**

And finish with *'Getting Better'* for **'The Back'**

OR

Complete all the *'Improving'* sections or all the *'Getting Better'* sections

OR

Make up your own!

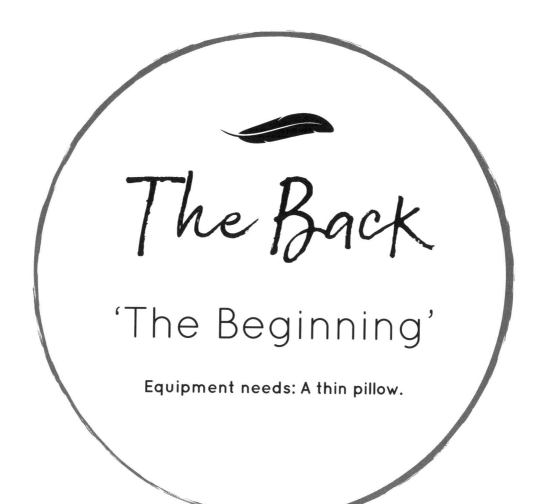

The Back

'The Beginning'

Equipment needs: A thin pillow.

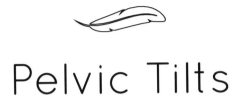

Pelvic Tilts

- Lie on your back with your knees bent and your feet hip socket distance apart.

- You might like to place a thin pillow under your head.

- You should find that there is a small gap underneath your lower back in your starting position.

- *Inhale to prepare.*

  - **Exhale** and roll the pelvis so that your lower back presses into the floor.

  - **Inhale** and return to the starting position.

  - Repeat eight times.

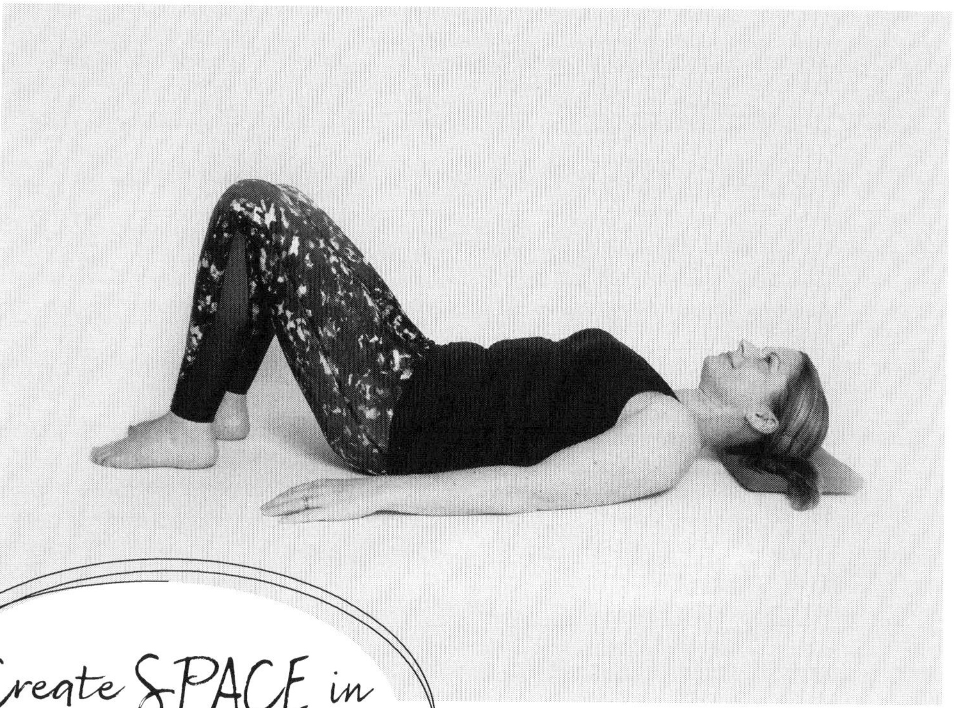

'Create SPACE in the lower back'

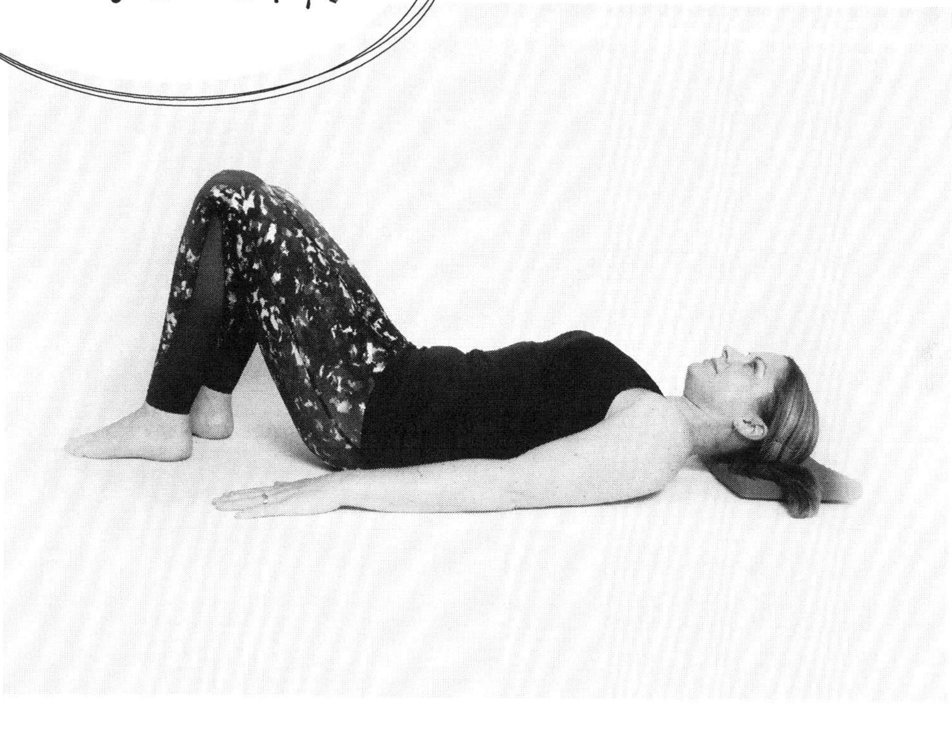

Side Rolls

From the same starting position as for Pelvic Tilts, take your arms out to the sides, palms up.

- **Inhale** to prepare.

- *Exhale and gently roll both legs to one side.*

    - Allow your head to turn to the opposite side.

    - Turn down the palm that you are looking at.

    - **Inhale** and hold the position.

    - **Exhale** to return to the start.

    - Repeat eight times on each side.

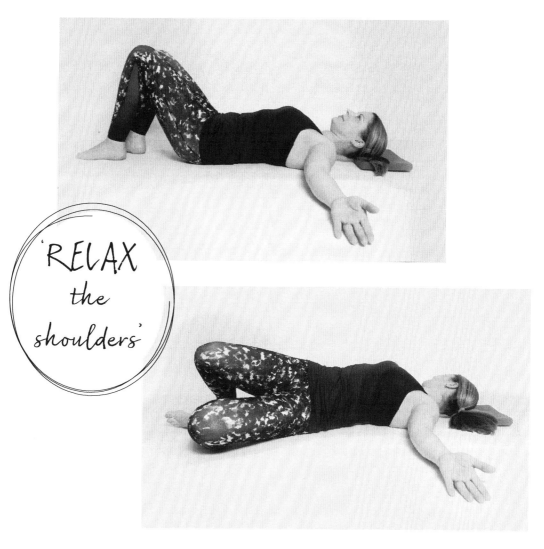

'RELAX
the
shoulders'

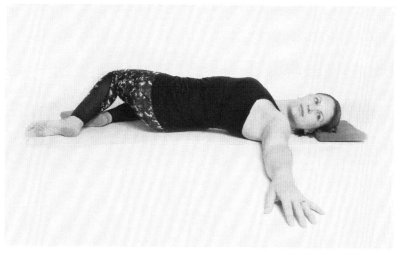

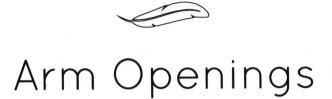

Arm Openings

- Lie on your side with a pillow under your head, arms outstretched and palms together.

- Bend the knees so that the feet are in line with the back of the body.

- **Inhale** to prepare.

- **Exhale** and trail the fingers of your top hand across your chest, following it with your eyes.

- Rotate your body from the ribcage, keep your knees together.

- Finish the action with the top arm outstretched on the other side of your body away from the floor.

- **Inhale** and hold this position.

- **Exhale** to return to the start.

- Repeat eight times on each side.

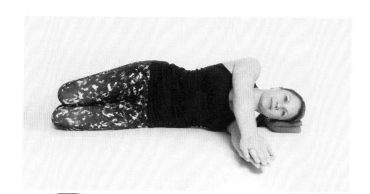

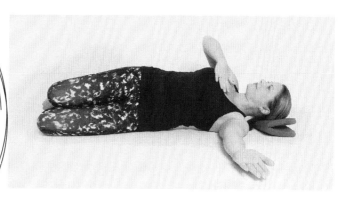

'Allow the ribcage to SOFTEN into the floor'

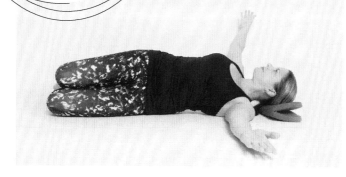

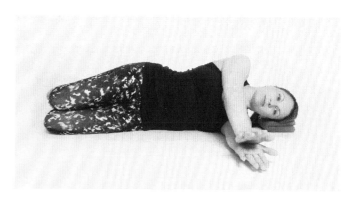

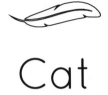

Cat

- Start on all fours, hands underneath the shoulders and knees underneath the hips.

- Allow the natural curves in your spine to sit comfortably.

- **Inhale** to prepare.

- **Exhale** and round the spine, pushing it towards the ceiling.

- Avoid gripping in your legs and buttocks.

Draw the abdominal muscles in tightly.

- **Inhale** and hold the position.

- **Exhale** to return to the start.

- Repeat eight times.

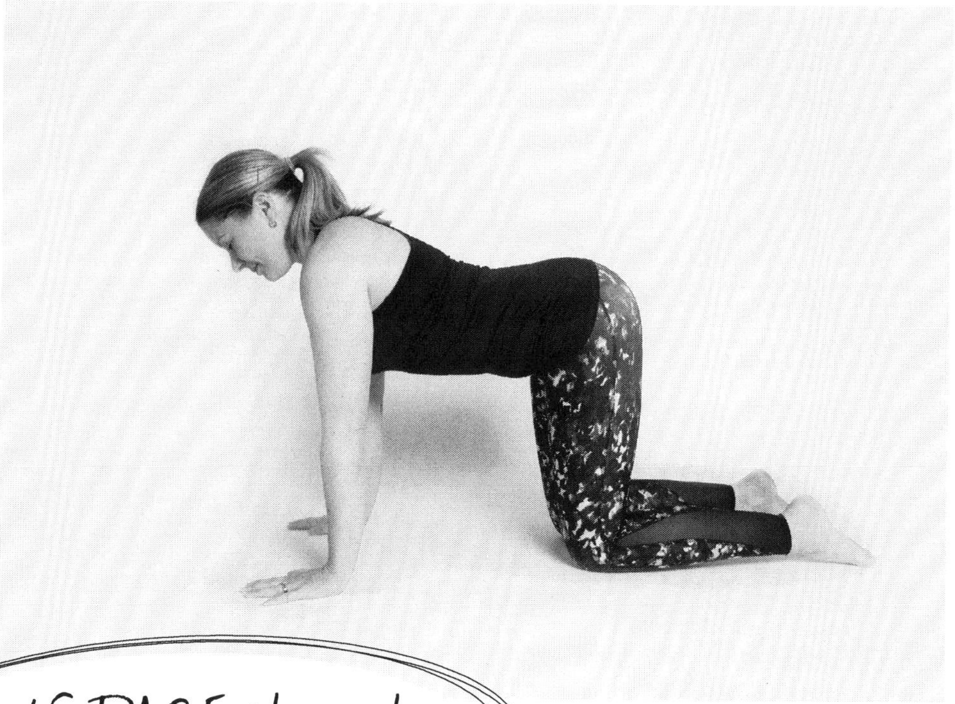

'Find SPACE through the back of the body'

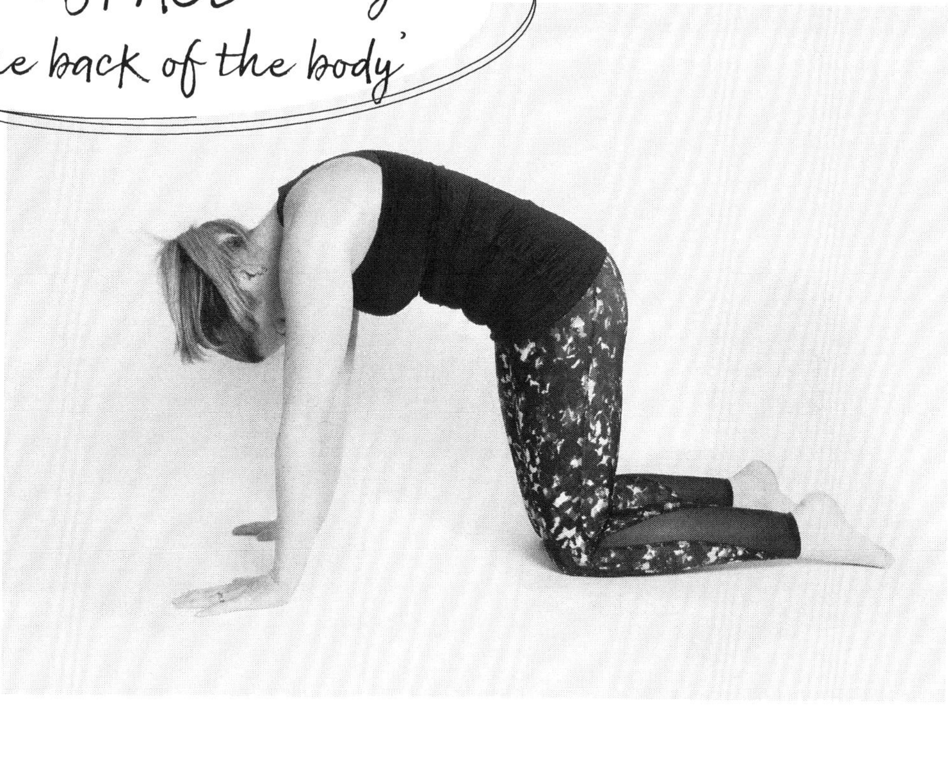

Half a Roll Down

- Stand with your knees softly bent, hands on the thighs.

- **Inhale** to lengthen through your spine.

- **Exhale** and gently peel the spine downwards bone by bone, starting with the head.

- *Allow your hands to slide down your legs.*

  - When you have gone as far as you feel comfortable with, **inhale** and hold.

  - **Exhale** to roll back up.

  - Repeat eight times.

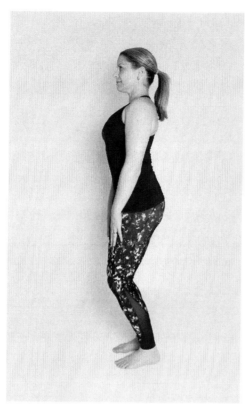

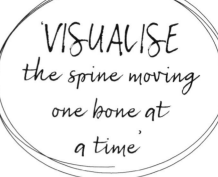

'VISUALISE
the spine moving
one bone at
a time'

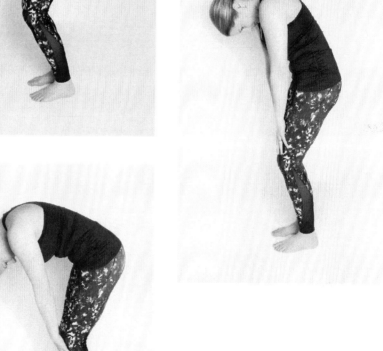

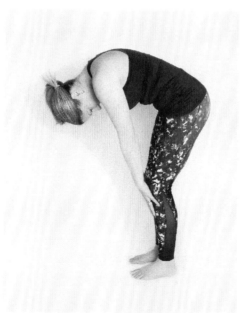

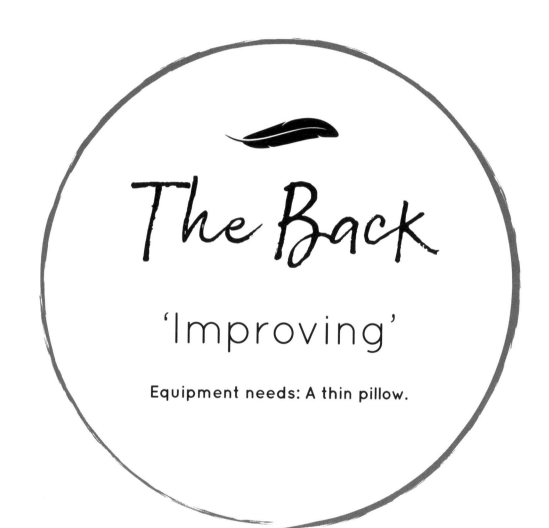

The Back

'Improving'

Equipment needs: A thin pillow.

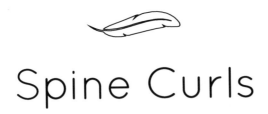

Spine Curls

From your Pelvic Tilts starting position:

- **Inhale** to prepare.

    - **Exhale** and pin your lower back into the floor.

    - Squeeze your buttocks, continue to exhale and peel the spine away from the floor one bone at a time.

    - **Inhale** in your highest position.

    - **Exhale** to roll the spine back to the starting position, with control.

    - Repeat eight times.

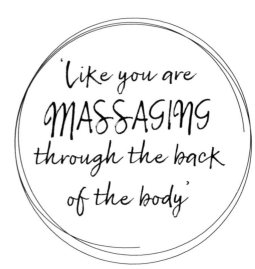

'Like you are MASSAGING through the back of the body'

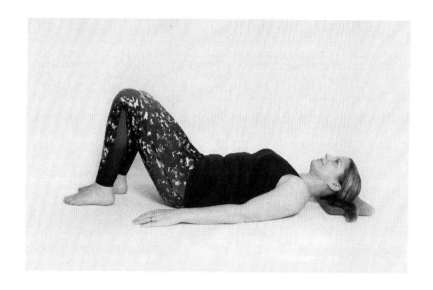

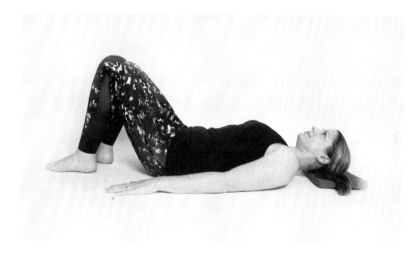

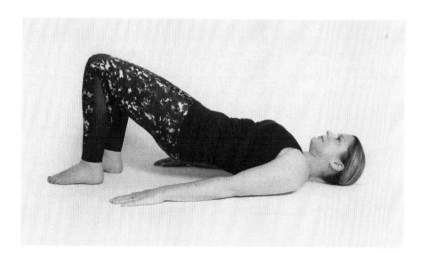

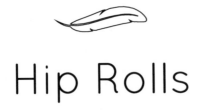

Hip Rolls

- Stay lying on your back with the knees bent, but bring the feet and knees together.

- Take your arms out to the sides, palms up (as for Side Rolls).

- **Inhale** to prepare.

- **Exhale** and drop the knees and pelvis to one side, trying to keep the legs together.

- *The legs may not go to the floor.*

  - Turn your head to the opposite side.

  - Turn down the palm that you are looking at.

  - **Inhale** and hold.

  - **Exhale** to return to the start.

  - Repeat eight times on each side.

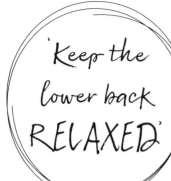

'Keep the lower back RELAXED'

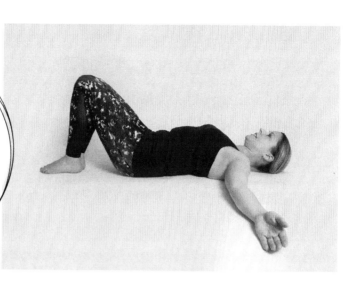

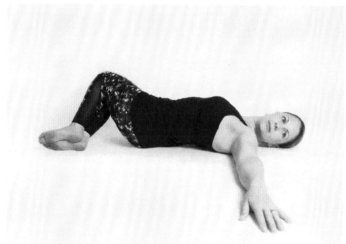

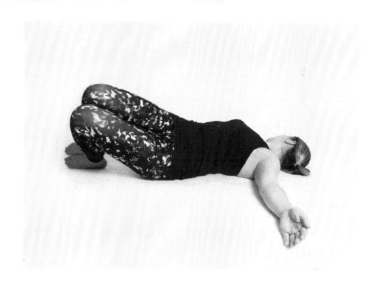

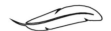

Cat (plus Extension)

- Start on all fours, hands underneath the shoulders and knees underneath the hips.

- Allow the natural curves in your spine to sit comfortably.

- **Inhale** to prepare.

- **Exhale** and round the spine, pushing it towards the ceiling.

- Avoid gripping in your legs and buttocks.

- Draw the abdominal muscles in tightly.

- **Inhale** and hold the position.

- **Exhale** to return to the start.

Optional:

- **Inhale** and tip the spine in the other direction, drop the belly towards the floor and send the chest forwards through the shoulders.

- **Exhale** and head off back in the direction of the ceiling again.

- Repeat eight times.

'As if you are WAVING the spine'

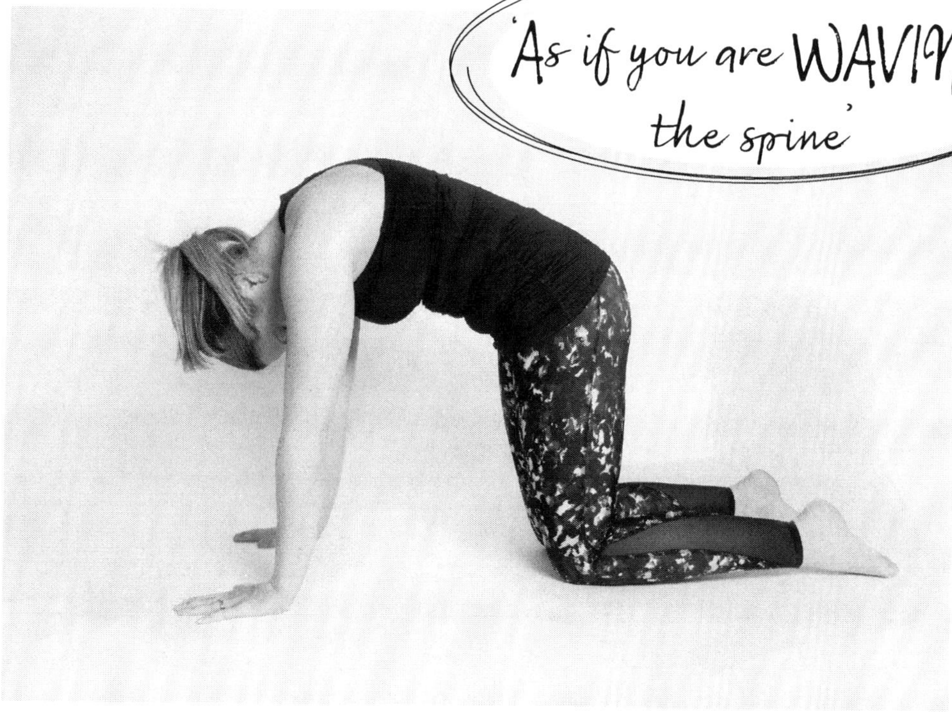

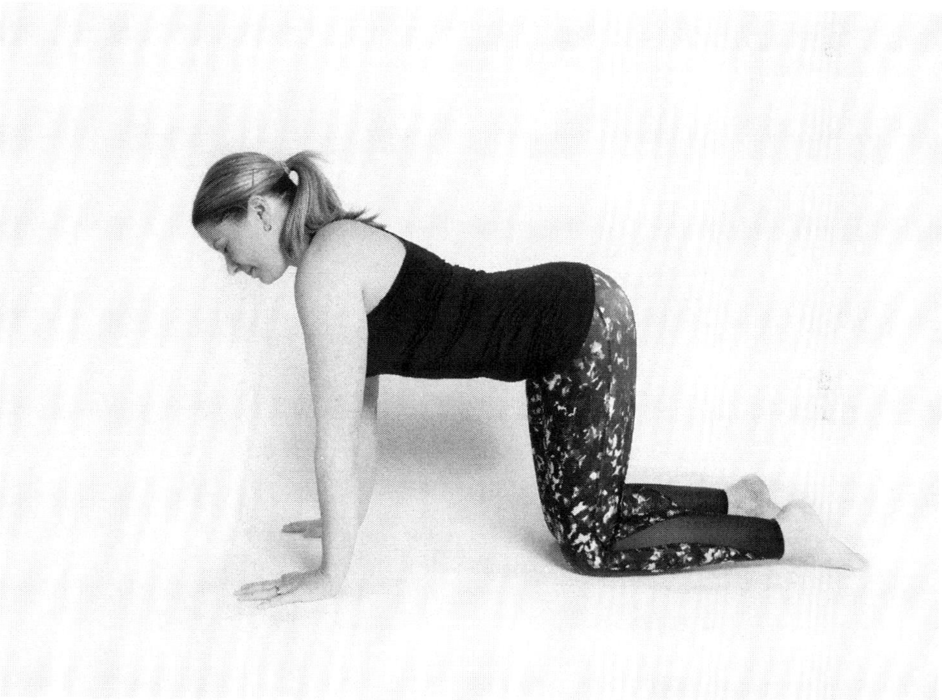

Threading the Needle

From your 'all fours' starting position:

- **Inhale** to prepare.

- **Exhale** and slide one hand along the floor, underneath the supporting arm.

- **Inhale** and reach the arm further.

- **Exhale** to return to the start.

- **Repeat** eight times on each side.

'AIM to keep your ear in line with your supporting hand's thumb'

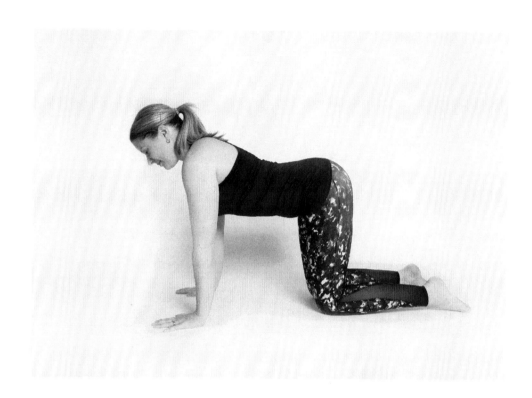

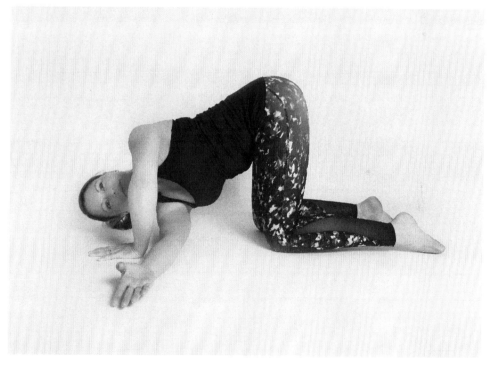

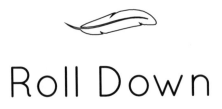

Roll Down

- Stand with your knees straight but not locked, arms down by your sides.

- **Inhale** to lengthen through your spine.

- **Exhale** and gently peel the spine downwards bone by bone, starting with the head.

- Allow your arms to hang gently in front of you.

- When you have gone as far as you feel comfortable with, **inhale** and hold.

- **Exhale** to roll back up.

- Repeat eight times.

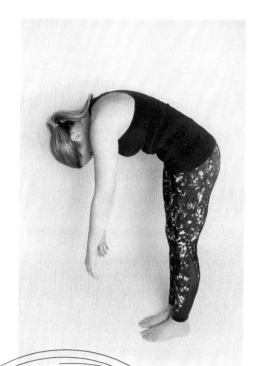

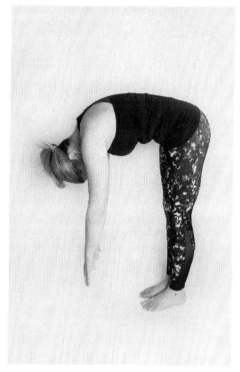

'PEEL the spine away from an imaginary surface'

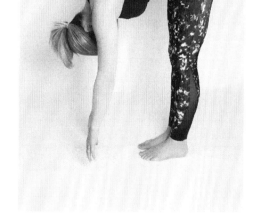

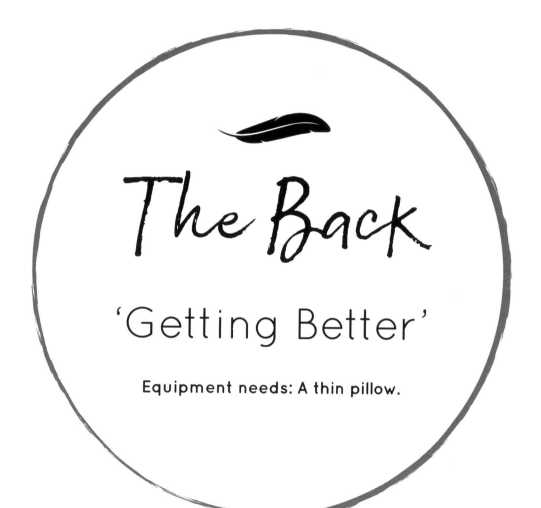

The Back

'Getting Better'

Equipment needs: A thin pillow.

Spine Curls plus Arms

From your Pelvic Tilts starting position:

- **Inhale** to prepare.

- **Exhale** and pin your lower back into the floor.

- Squeeze your buttocks, continue to exhale and peel the spine away from the floor one bone at a time.

- **Inhale** in your top position, taking the arms over your head to a point where you can still see the elbows.

- **Exhale** to roll the spine back to the starting position, with control.

- **Inhale** to return the arms to the sides of your body.

- Repeat eight times.

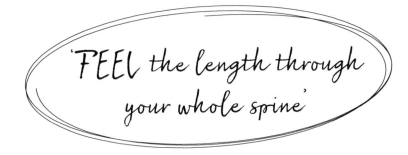

'FEEL the length through your whole spine'

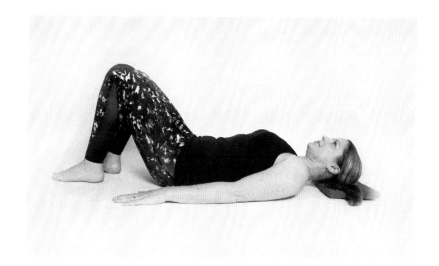

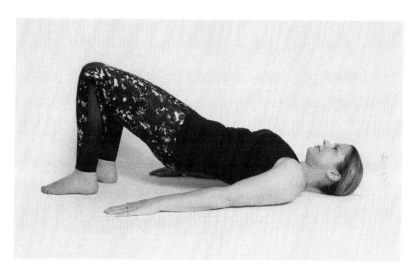

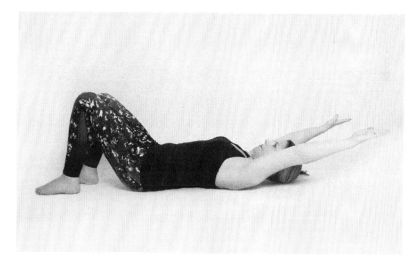

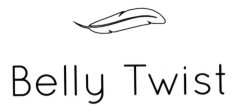

Belly Twist

- Stay lying on your back with the knees bent, but bring the feet and knees together.

- Lift the legs away from the floor so that the hips and knees are at a 90-degree angle.

- Take your arms out to the sides, palms up (as for Side Rolls and Hip Rolls).

- **Inhale** to prepare.

- **Exhale** and drop the knees and pelvis to one side, trying to keep the legs together.

- *The legs may not go to the floor.*

- Turn your head to the opposite side.

- Turn down the palm that you are looking at.

- **Inhale** and hold.

- **Exhale** to return to the start.

Optional:

- Hold the position for four breath rounds, repeating twice on each side.

OR

- Repeat eight times on each side.

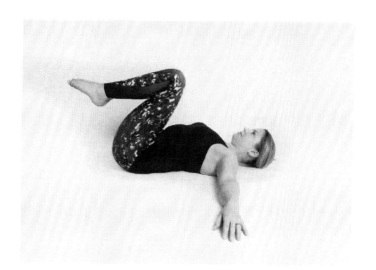

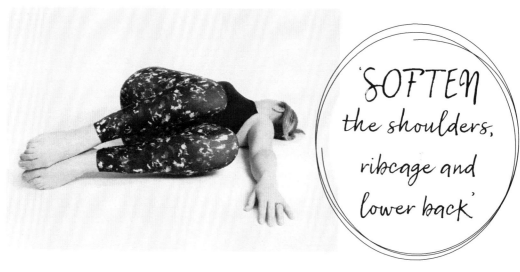

'SOFTEN the shoulders, ribcage and lower back'

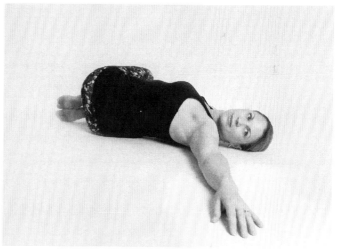

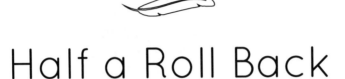

Half a Roll Back

- Start sitting tall with your knees bent, heels digging into the floor and arms outstretched in front.

- **Inhale** to lengthen the spine.

- **Exhale** and roll the pelvis underneath you and backwards, as if you are trying to get your lower back to touch the floor.

- *Pull the abdominal muscles in tightly.*

  - **Inhale** and hold the position.

  - **Exhale** to roll back up to sitting.

  - Repeat eight times.

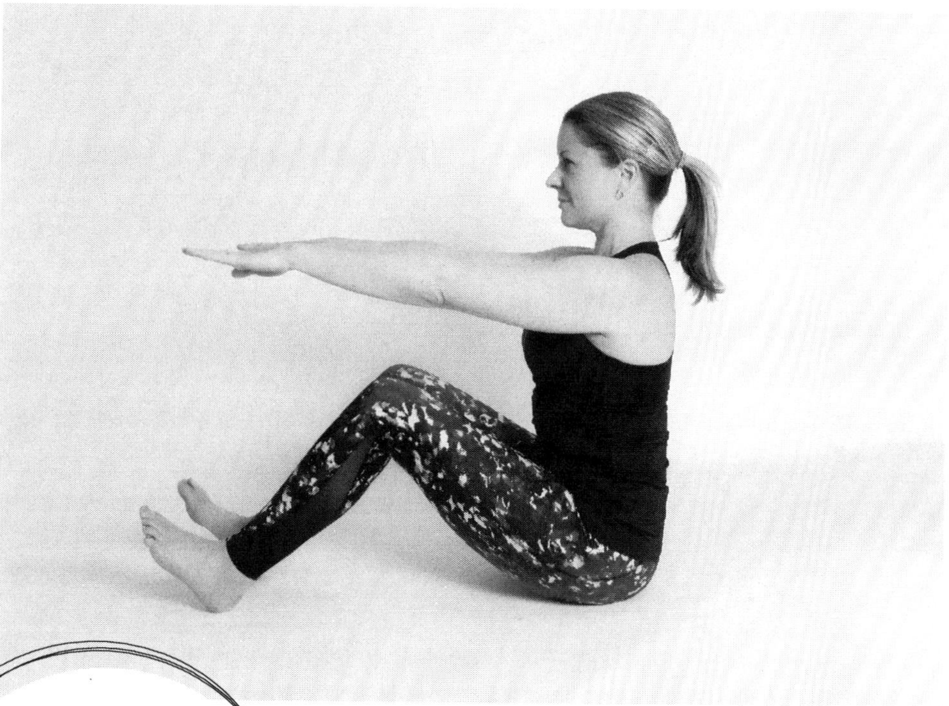

'RELAX the hips and thighs'

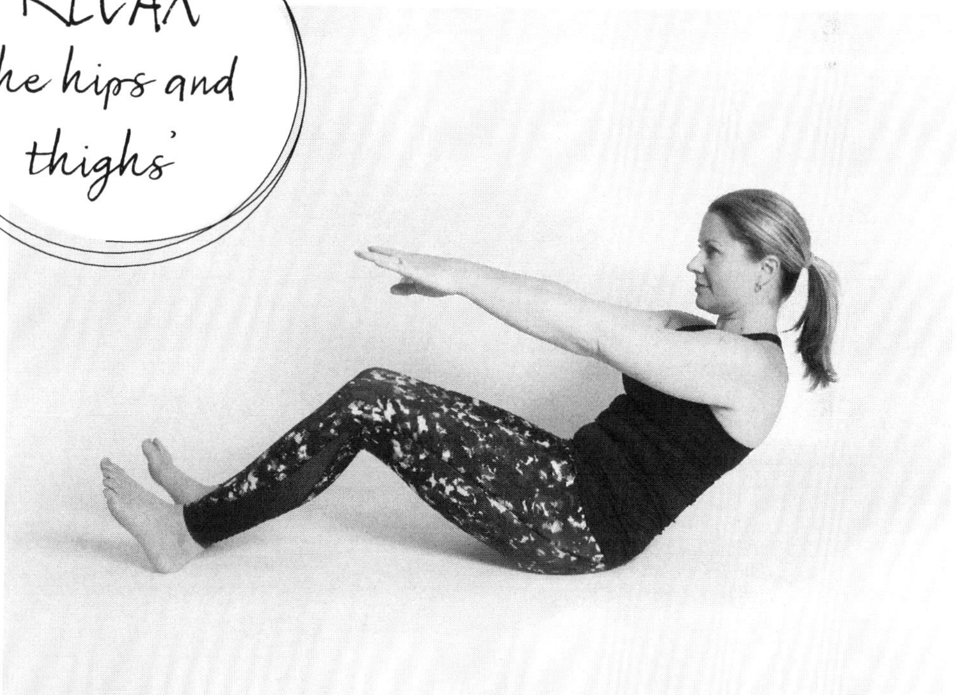

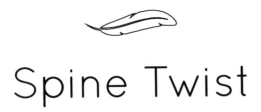

Spine Twist

- From your seated position (legs bent or straight or sitting on a wedge/block) stretch your arms out to the sides.

- **Exhale** to prepare.

- **Inhale** to rotate your body and arms in one direction.

- **Exhale** return to the centre.

- Repeat eight times on each side.

'FEEL
the length in
the spine'

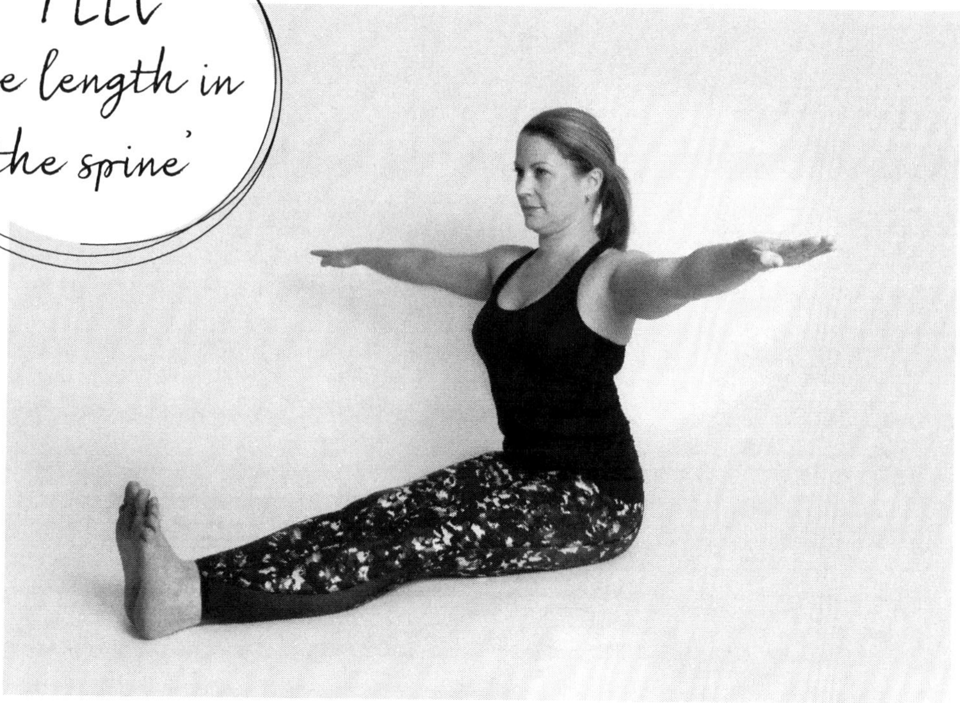

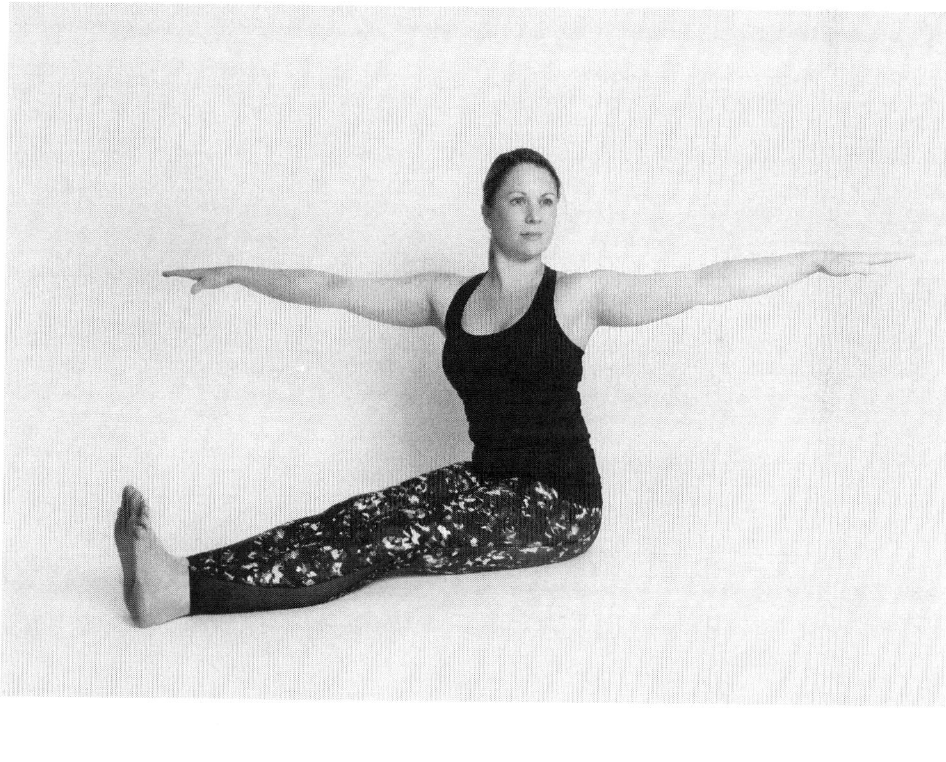

Upper Back Extension

Also useful for *'Improving'* **The Shoulders**

- Lie on your front with your hands flat either side of your face, elbows down.

- **Inhale** to prepare.

- **Exhale** and peel the upper body away from the mat, as far as your lower ribs.

- **Inhale** to lower back down.

- Repeat eight times.

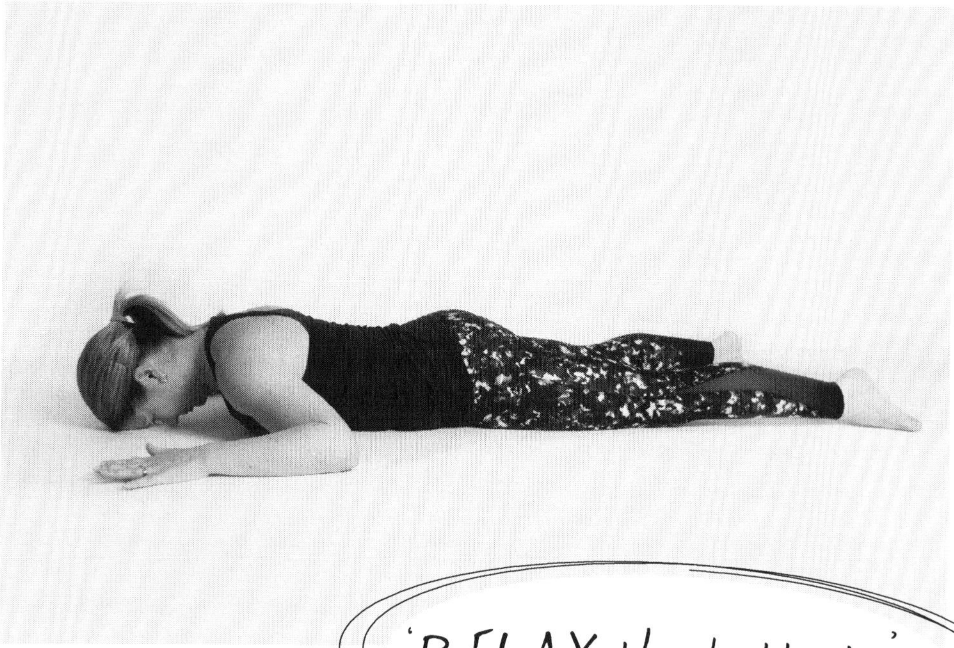

'RELAX the buttocks'

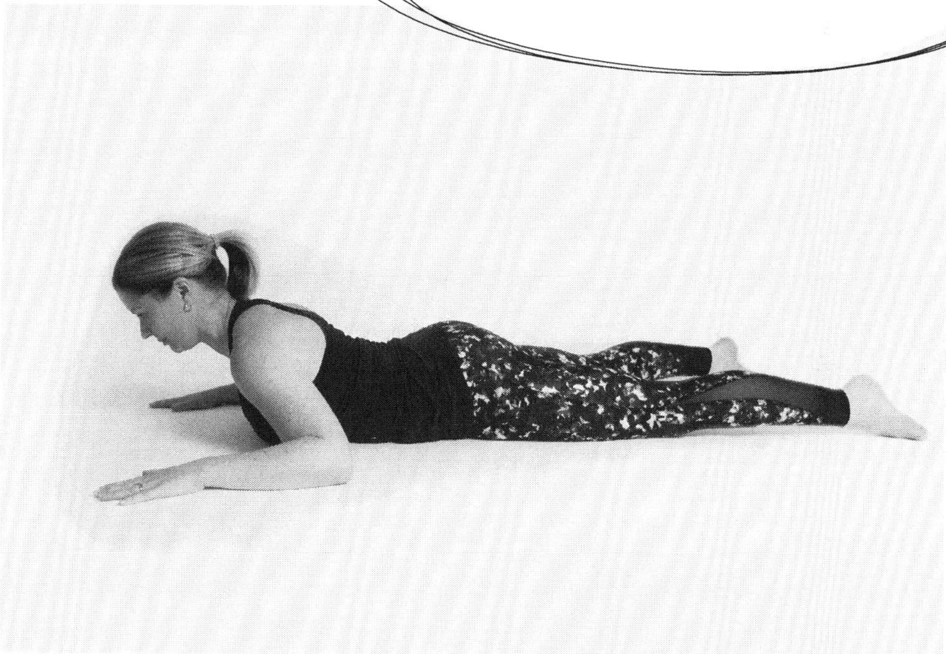

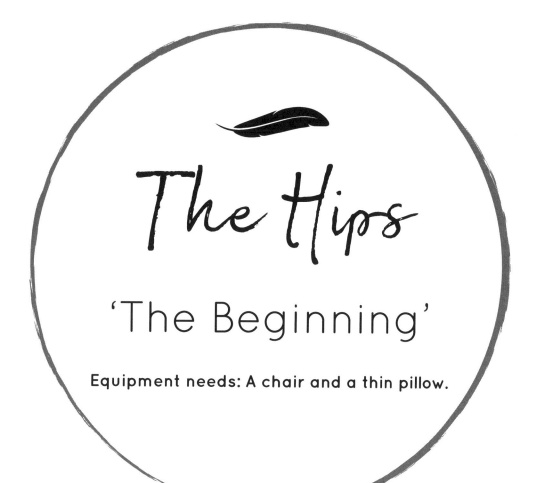

The Hips

'The Beginning'

Equipment needs: A chair and a thin pillow.

Knee Drops

- Lie on your back with your feet hip socket distance apart.

- Place the thin pillow under the back of your head.

- **Inhale** to prepare.

- **Exhale** to drop one knee out to the side (on to the side of the foot).

- *It should go to about 45 degrees before the pelvis moves.*

- Keep the pelvis centred.

- **Inhale** to return the leg to the centre.

- **Exhale** to repeat on the other side.

- Repeat eight times on each side.

'IMAGINE the middle of the pelvis is anchored to the floor'

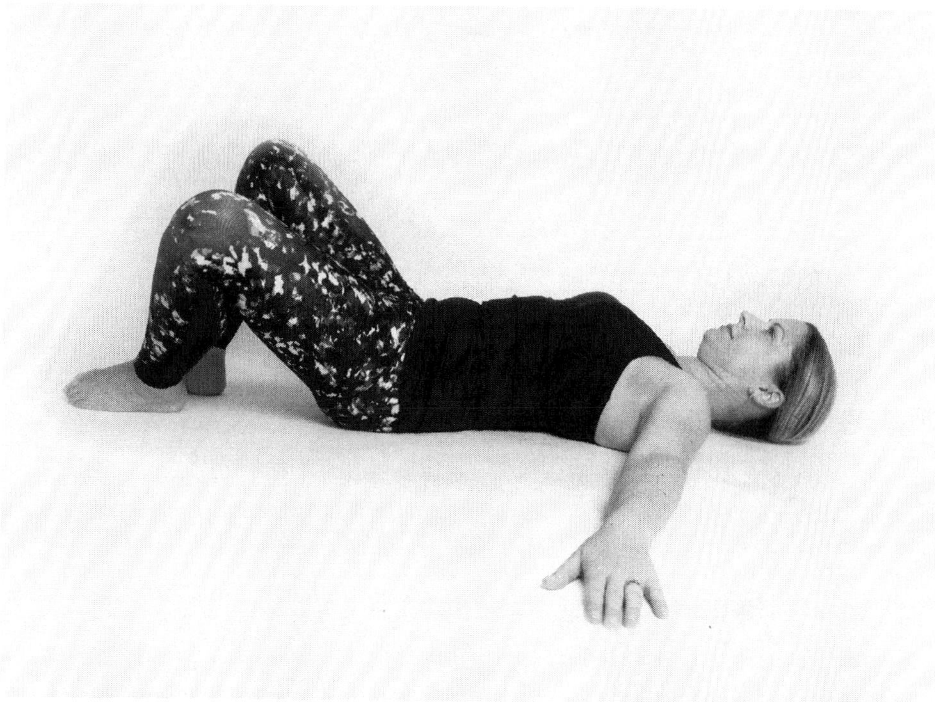

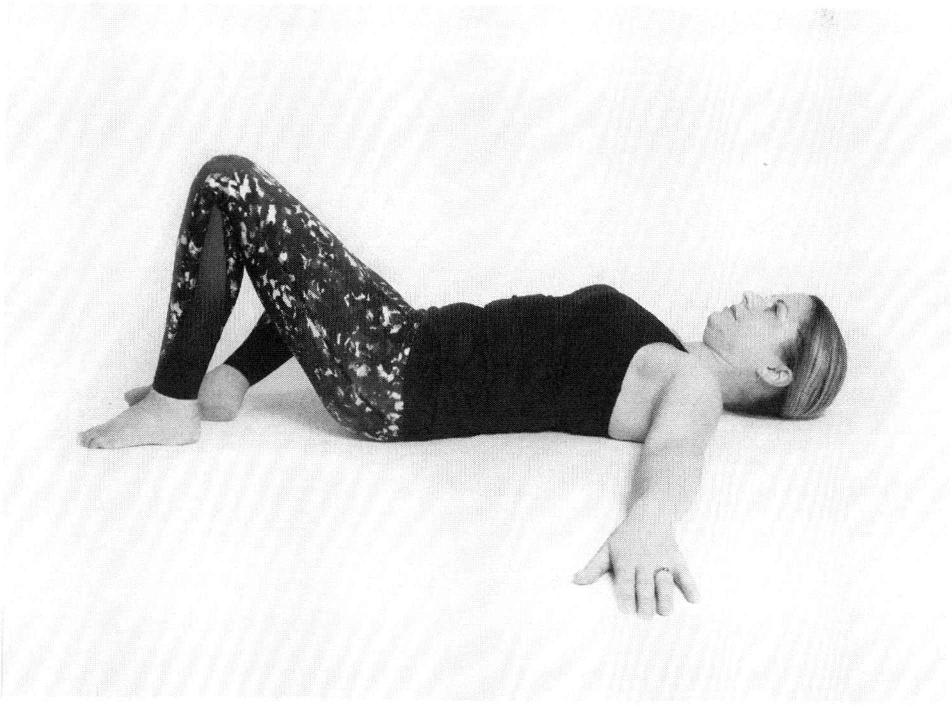

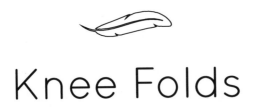

Knee Folds

From your previous starting position in Knee Drops:

- **Inhale** to prepare.

- **Exhale** and slowly bring one leg up to a 90-degree angle at the hip and knee.

- Draw the abdominals in tightly.

- **Inhale** and slowly lower the leg back to the floor.

- *Keep the ribs glued to the mat and the pelvis steady.*

- Repeat eight times on each side.

'As if you are moving through SYRUP'

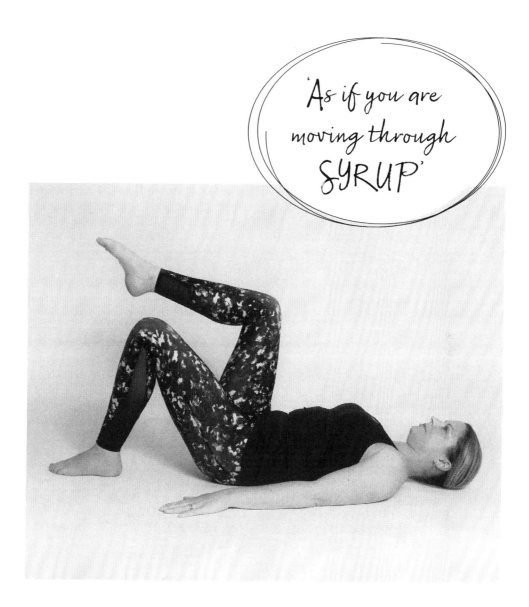

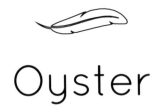

Oyster

- Lie on your side with your head resting on an outstretched arm (optional to put the thin pillow between the arm and the ear).

- One hand supports firmly, in front of the body.

- Line the feet up with the spine, knees bent.

- *Feet need to be slightly off the floor, knees down.*

- **Inhale** to prepare.

- **Exhale** and keep the feet together as you lift open the top knee.

- *Use the supporting hand to help push the knee a little further out if possible.*

- **Inhale** to lower back down to the starting position.

- Repeat eight times on each side.

'Stay SECURE through your supporting hand'

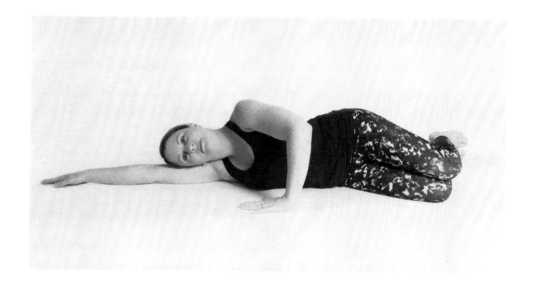

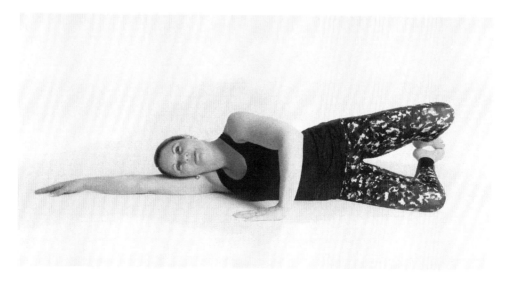

Prone Leg Lift

- Lie on your front with your head resting on your hands.

- **Inhale** to prepare.

- **Exhale** and squeeze your buttocks to anchor the pelvis and lift one straight leg away from the floor.

- *If your pelvis is steady, you will not lift very high.*

- **Inhale** and lower the leg.

- Repeat eight times on each side.

'FEEL the heaviness of your pelvis'

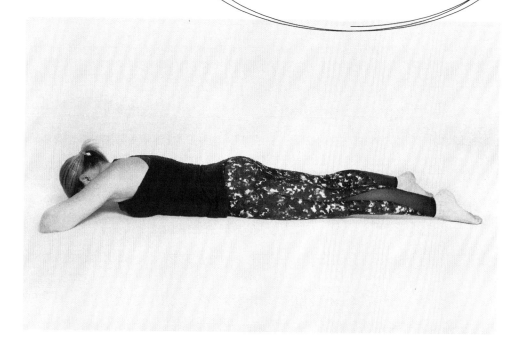

Standing Leg Swings

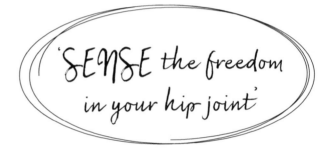

'SENSE the freedom in your hip joint'

- Stand side on to the back of a chair so that you can hold on for support.

- **Inhale** and lengthen through the spine.

- *Take your weight into one leg.*

- **Exhale** and swing your free leg gently forwards.

- **Inhale** to swing it backwards.

- Repeat eight times on each leg.

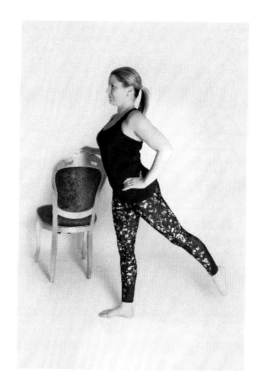
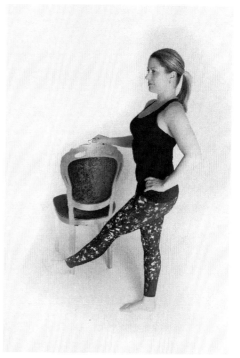
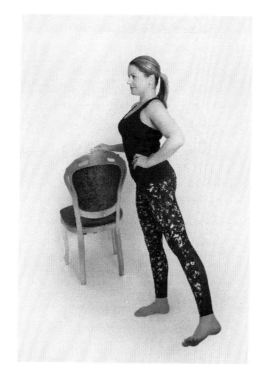

The Hips

'Improving'

Equipment needs: A bit of stretch band
or a belt/scarf. A thin pillow.

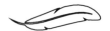

Hamstrings Stretch

- Lie on your back with your band/belt/scarf around one foot and the thin pillow under your head.

- Stretch that leg up towards the ceiling and keep the other knee bent.

- *Try to keep the tailbone anchored to the floor.*

- **Inhale** and **exhale** eight times as you hold the stretch.

- Change legs and repeat.

'LENGTHEN both up to the ceiling and down through the back of the pelvis'

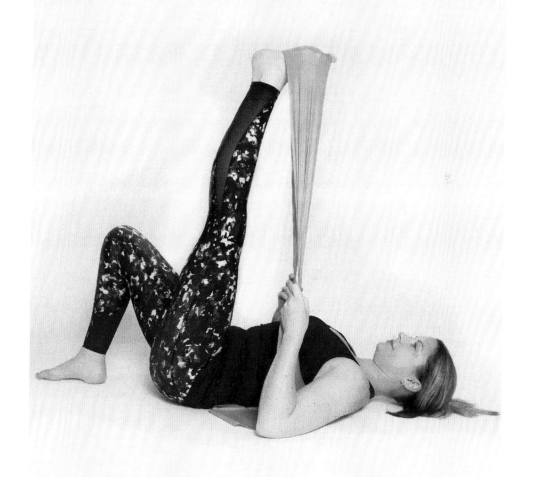

Knee Circles

- From your previous starting position in Hamstrings Stretch, lift one leg until the hip and knee are both at 90 degrees.

- **Inhale** to complete one full rotation of the thigh bone in the hip socket.

- **Exhale** to complete the next full rotation.

- *Try to keep the pelvis still.*

- Repeat in this manner until you have done eight in each direction.

- Change legs and repeat.

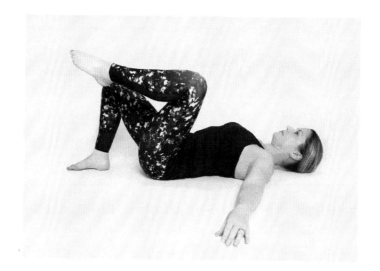

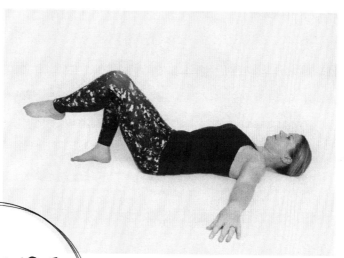

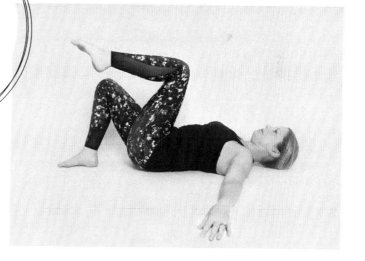

'VISUALISE a pestle and mortar'

Oyster/Charleston

- Lie on your side (as for Oyster).

- **Inhale** to prepare.

- **Exhale** and lift the top knee, using the supporting hand to achieve further range.

- **Inhale** and now bring the knees together taking the feet apart.

- **Exhale** to bring the feet back together, knees apart.

- Repeat eight times on each side.

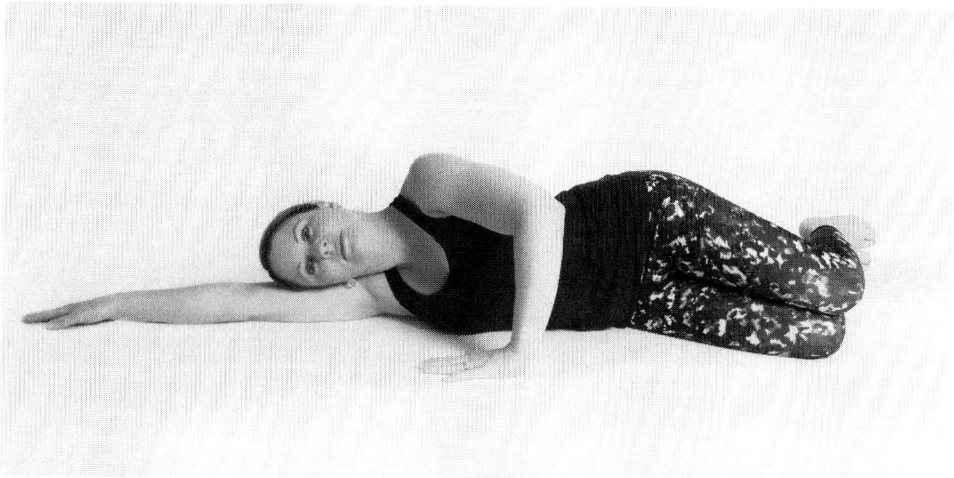

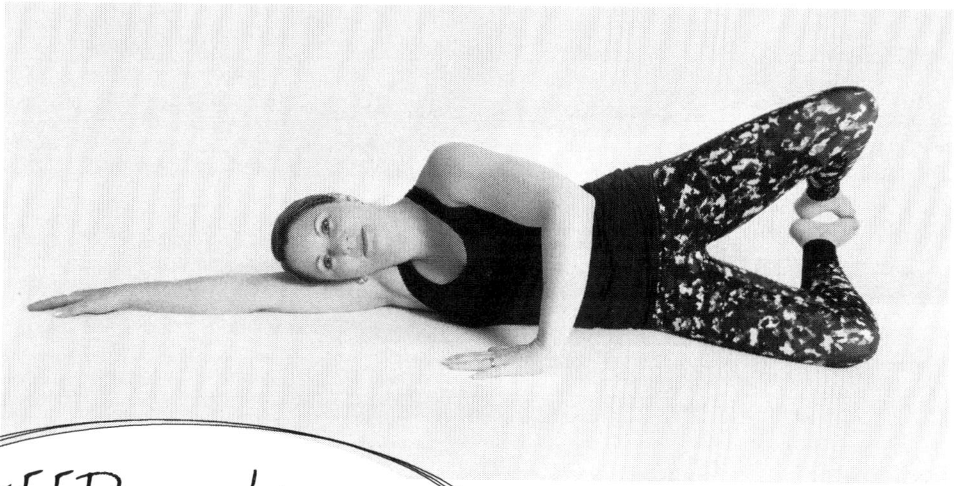

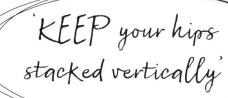

'KEEP your hips stacked vertically'

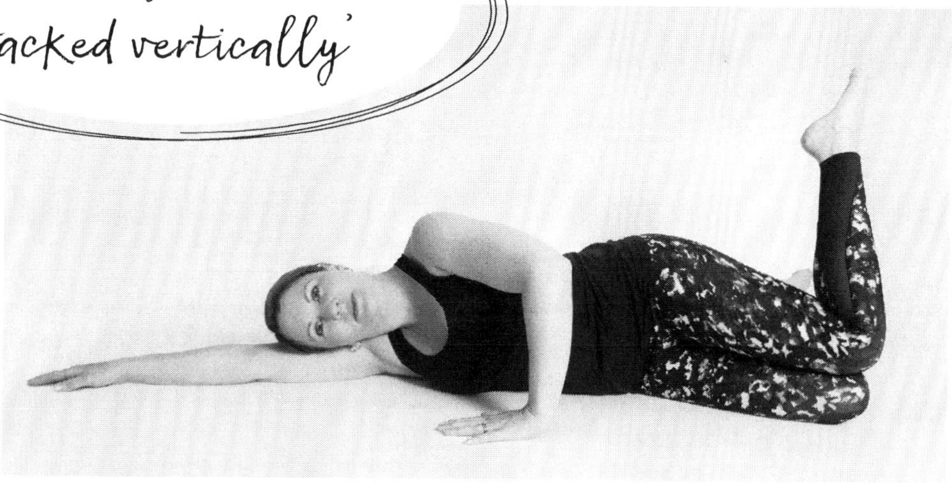

Single Leg Kick

- Lie on your front with your head resting on your hands.

- **Inhale** to lift a straight leg away from the floor, squeezing the buttocks.

- **Exhale** to bend the knee, bringing the foot towards the buttock.

- *Aim to keep both the hips level against the floor and the knees fairly close together.*

- Repeat eight times on each side.

'ANCHOR both sides of the pelvis to the floor'

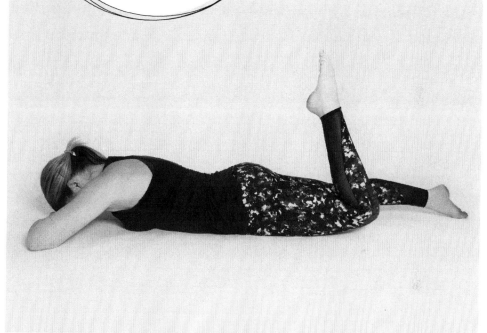

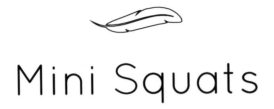

Mini Squats

Also useful for *'Improving'* **The Knees**

- Stand tall and balanced on both feet.

- **Inhale** to lengthen the spine.

- **Exhale** and bend the knees, sending them forwards rather than together or out to the sides.

- *Keep the weight balanced on your feet.*

- Repeat eight times.

'TRACK
the knees in
line with your
second toe'

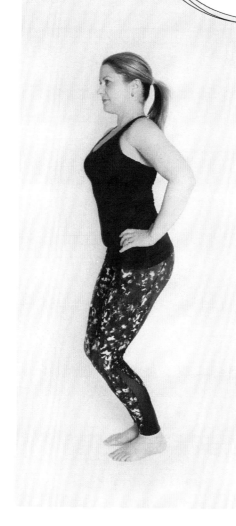
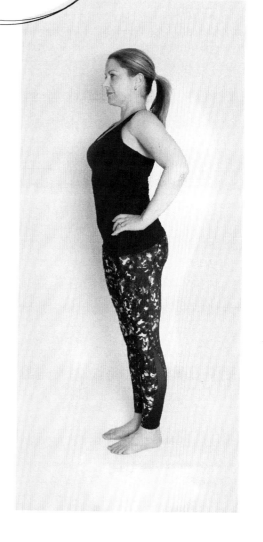

The Hips

'Getting Better'

Equipment needs: A bit of stretch band
or a belt/scarf. A thin pillow.

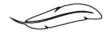

Hamstrings to Hip Stretch

- Lie on your back with a thin pillow under your head.

- Put one foot in your band/belt/scarf.

- Stretch your other leg out along the floor and slightly out to the side.

- **Inhale** and **exhale** eight times as you hold first the Hamstrings Stretch.

- **Inhale** and **exhale** eight times as you hold the leg across the body towards your opposite shoulder.

- Repeat on both sides.

'WORK into your edges'

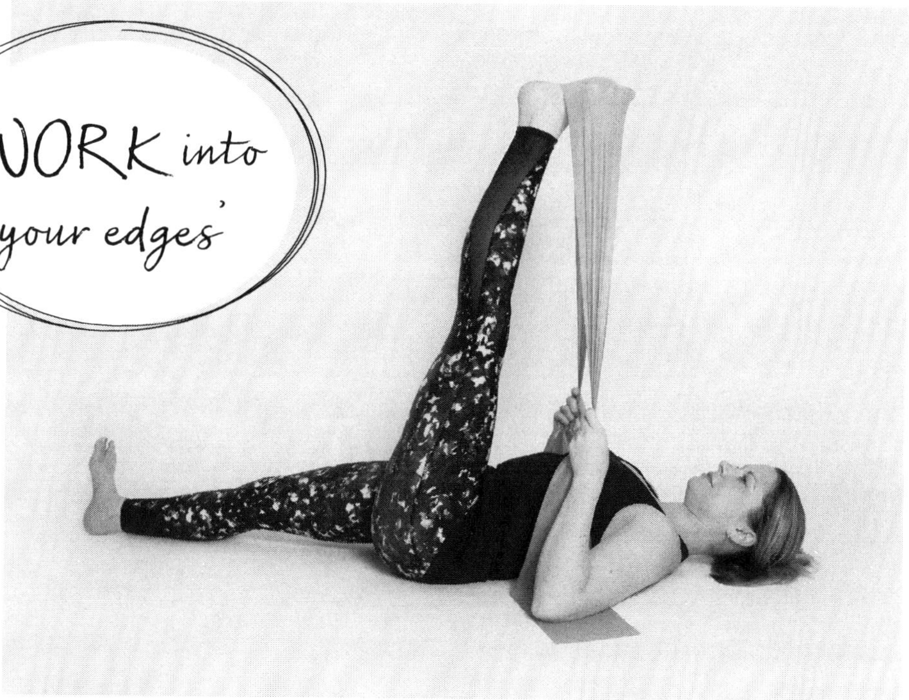

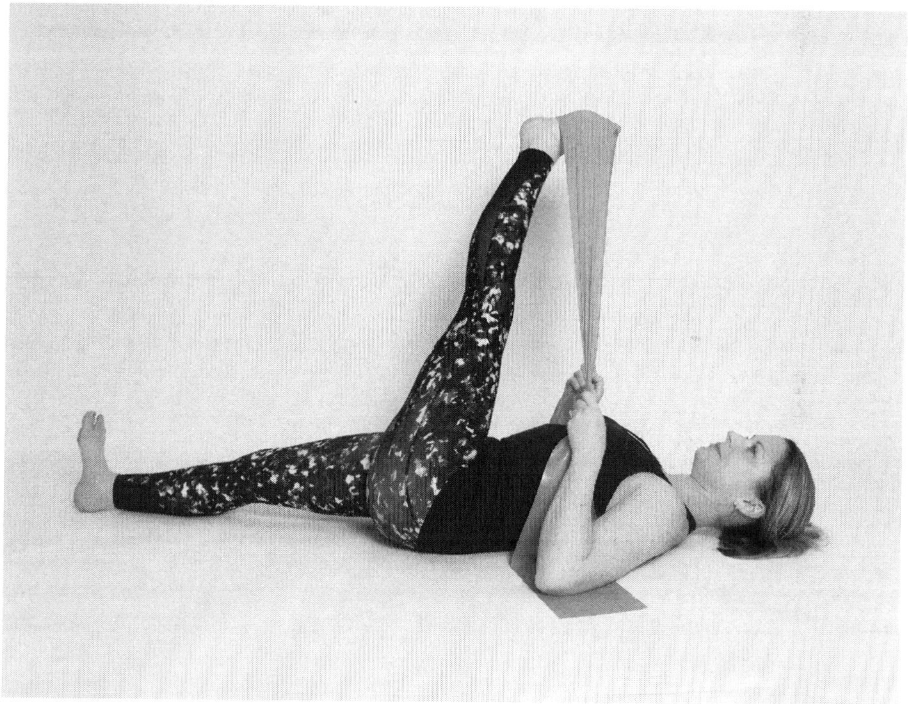

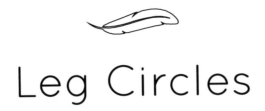

Leg Circles

MAINTAIN the stability of your pelvis'

From your starting position for Hamstrings to Hip Stretch:

- **Inhale** as you move the leg first across towards the opposite shoulder.

- **Exhale** and complete one full circle of the leg in the hip joint.

- *Keep the pelvis steady.*

- Repeat eight times in each direction on each leg.

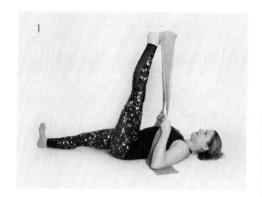

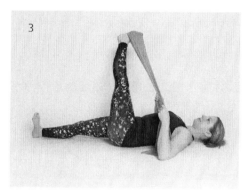

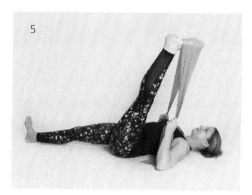

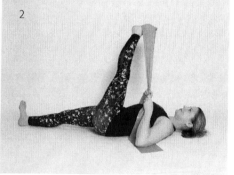

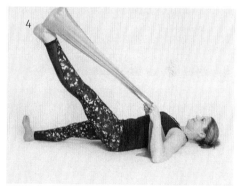

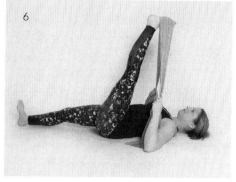

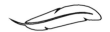

Side Lying Leg Series

1) Abduction

- Lie on your side with your head resting on an outstretched arm (optional to put the thin pillow between the arm and the ear).

- One hand supports firmly, in front of the body.

- The bottom leg bends to 90 degrees.

- The top leg stretches out in line with the spine.

- **Inhale** to prepare.

- **Exhale** and lift the top leg as high as it will go without shortening in the waist and/or rotating from the hip.

- **Inhale** to lower.

- Repeat eight times and follow with Forward and Back.

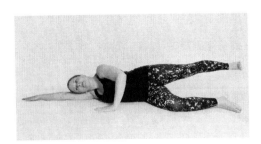
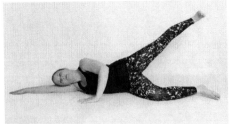

'FEEL the length in your working leg'

2) Forward and Back

- Start in the same position as for Abduction.

- **Inhale** to prepare.

- **Exhale** to take the straight leg forwards with flexed foot (push the heel away).

- **Inhale** to take it backwards and open up through the front of the hip.

- *Keep the hips stable.*

- Repeat eight times.

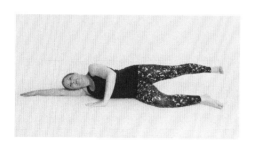
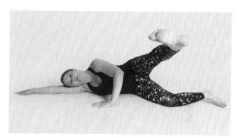
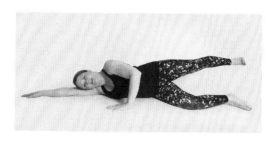

Double Leg Kick

- Lie on your front with your head resting on your hands.

- *Position the legs close together.*

  - **Inhale** to prepare, squeeze the buttocks and lift both legs away from the floor.

  - **Exhale** to bend the knees as if kicking both feet towards the buttocks.

  - *Try to keep your knees off the floor.*

  - **Inhale** and aim to lift the legs higher as you stretch them away, back to the floor.

  - Repeat eight times.

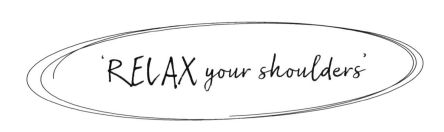

'RELAX your shoulders'

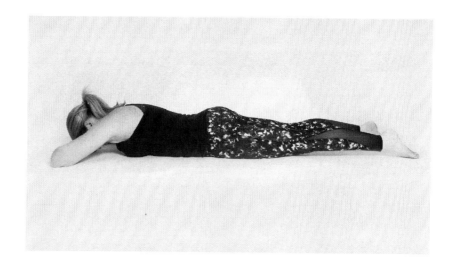

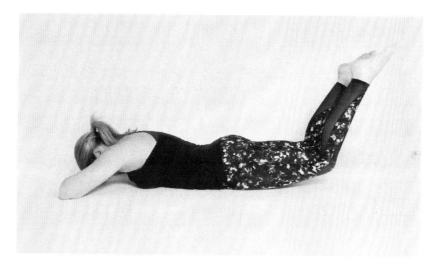

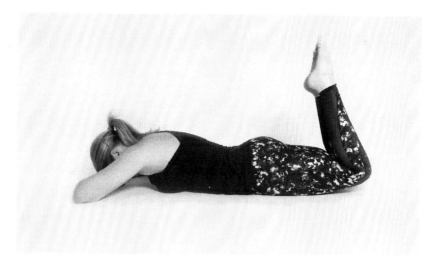

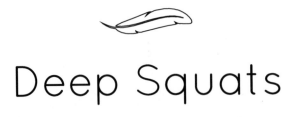

Deep Squats

Also useful for *'Getting Better'* **The Knees**

- Stand tall and balanced on both feet.

- **Inhale** to lengthen the spine.

- **Exhale** and bend the knees and hips as deeply as you feel comfortable.

- *Keep the weight balanced on your feet.*

- Repeat eight times.

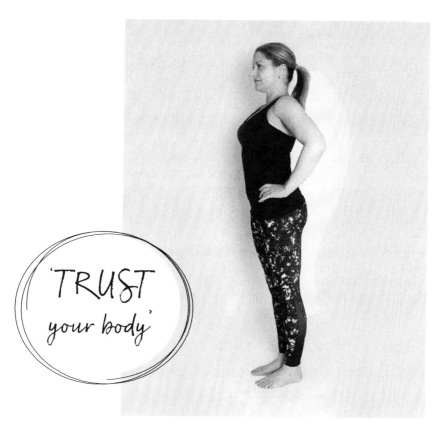

'TRUST
your body'

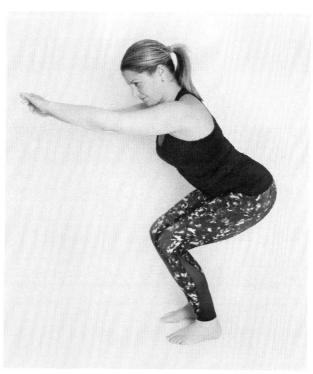

The Shoulders

'The Beginning'

Equipment needed: A wall and a (full) small water bottle.

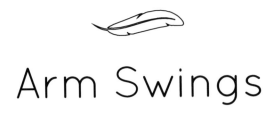

Arm Swings

- Stand tall with shoulders relaxed.

- **Inhale** to lengthen the spine and take both arms out in front of you.

- **Exhale** and swing one arm slowly downwards and behind you.

- **Inhale** to do the same on the other arm.

- Repeat eight times on each arm.

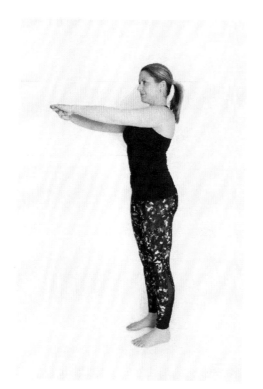

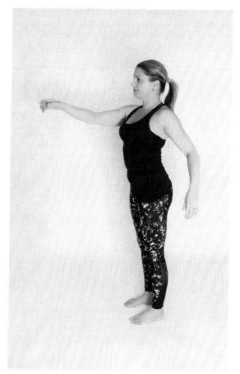

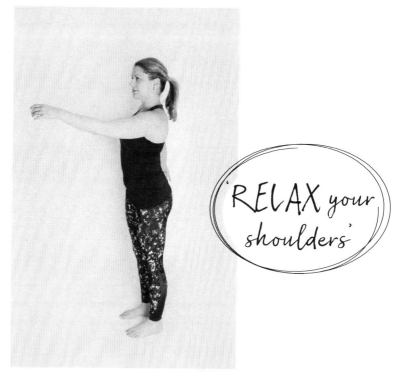

'RELAX your shoulders'

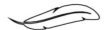

Walking Up a Wall

- Stand near a wall and place your fingers against it 'like a spider'.

- **Inhale** to lengthen the spine.

- **Exhale** and slowly start walking your hand as far up the wall as you can.

- **Inhale** to walk it back down.

- Repeat eight times on each arm.

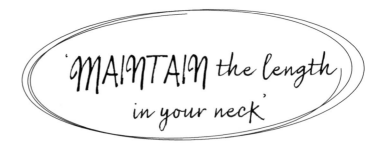

'MAINTAIN the length in your neck'

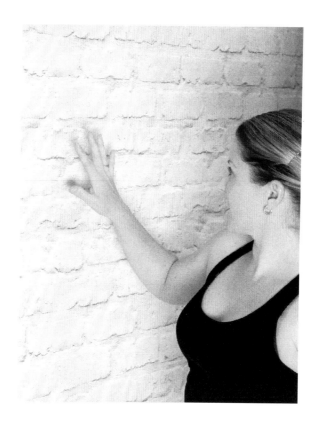

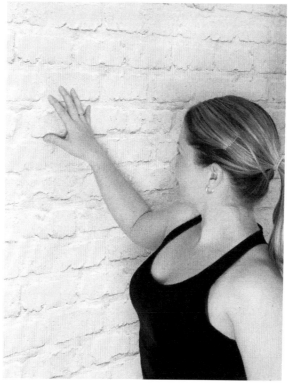

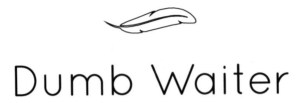

Dumb Waiter

- Stand tall and bend your elbows as if holding two bowls of soup in front of you.

- **Inhale** to lengthen the spine.

- **Exhale** to prepare.

- **Inhale** to open the arm up to the sides, rotating the upper arm bone in the shoulder joint.

- Repeat eight times.

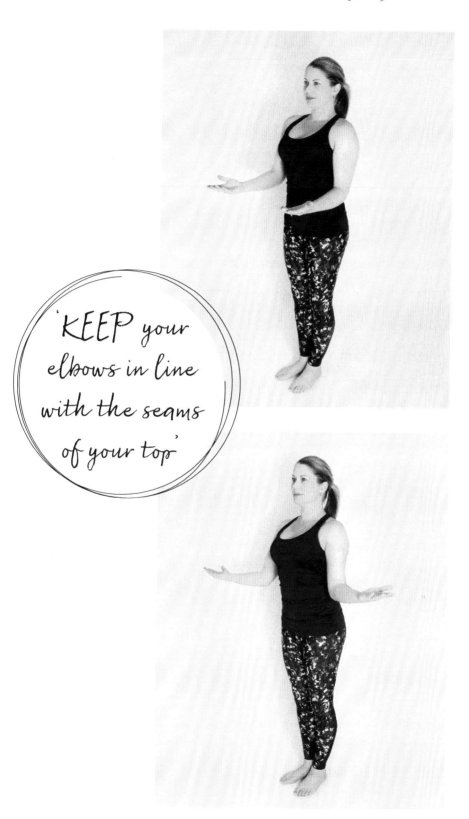

'KEEP your elbows in line with the seams of your top'

Hand Behind the Back

- Stand tall and hold your water bottle in one hand.

- **Inhale** to lengthen the spine.

- **Exhale** to pass the water bottle behind your back to the other hand.

- **Inhale** to take that arm out to the side.

- **Exhale** again to pass it back the other way.

- Keep passing from hand to hand and out to the sides eight times.

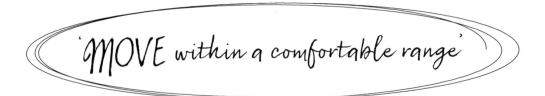

'*MOVE within a comfortable range*'

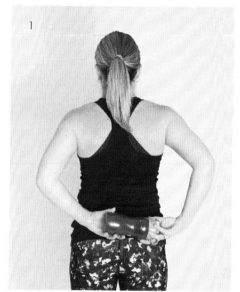

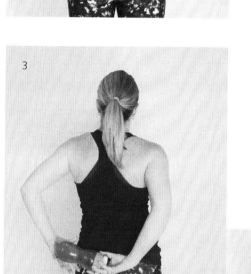

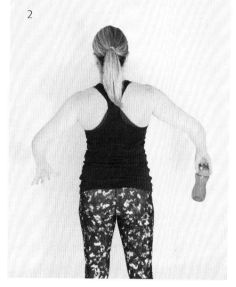

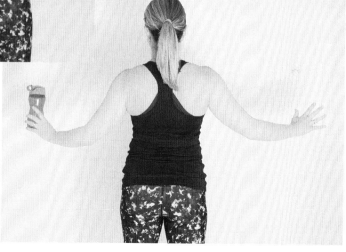

Small Arm Circles

- Stand slightly leaning forwards so that one arm hangs freely.

- *The other hand can rest on your thigh or knee.*

  - **Inhale** and secure your standing position.

  - **Exhale** and swing your arm in one small but full circular motion.

  - **Inhale** to do the next circle.

  - Repeat eight times in each direction on each arm.

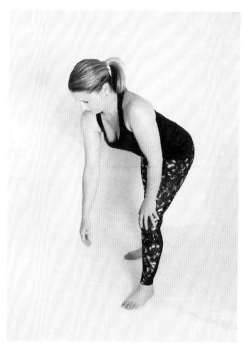

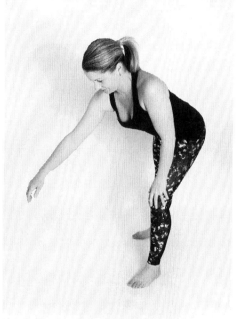

'FOCUS on release'

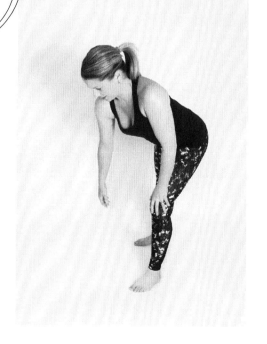

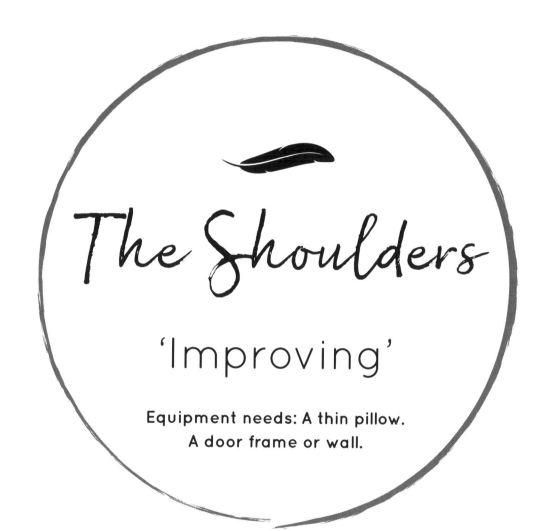

The Shoulders

'Improving'

Equipment needs: A thin pillow.
A door frame or wall.

Backstroke Arms

- Lie on your back with your feet hip socket distance apart.

- Place the thin pillow under the back of your head.

- **Inhale** to prepare.

- **Exhale** and take one arm over your head to a point where you can still see your elbow in your peripheral vision.

- **Inhale** to lift both arms up to vertical, ready for the changeover.

- **Exhale** to take the other arm over your head and the first arm down by your side.

- Repeat eight times on each arm.

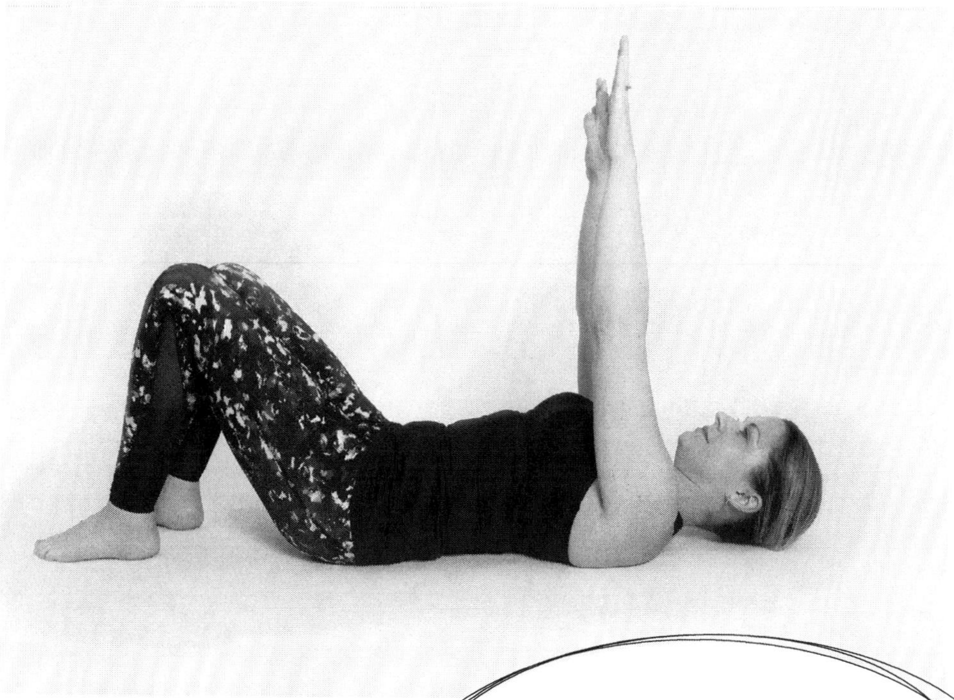

'ANCHOR your ribcage to the floor'

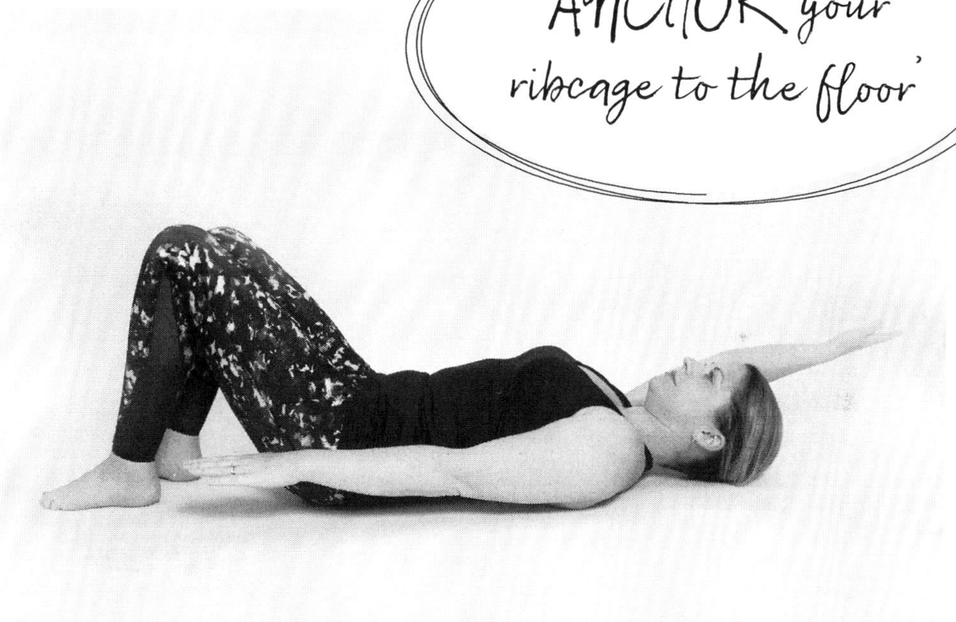

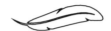

Door Frame/ Wall Stretch 1

- Place one hand on to a wall or against a door frame.

- Bend the elbow.

- Turn your body away from the arm.

- **Inhale** and **exhale** eight times as you hold the stretch.

- Repeat for eight breath rounds on the other side.

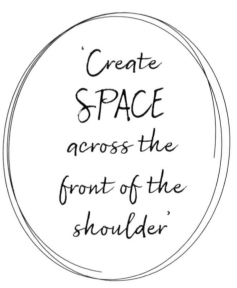

'Create SPACE across the front of the shoulder'

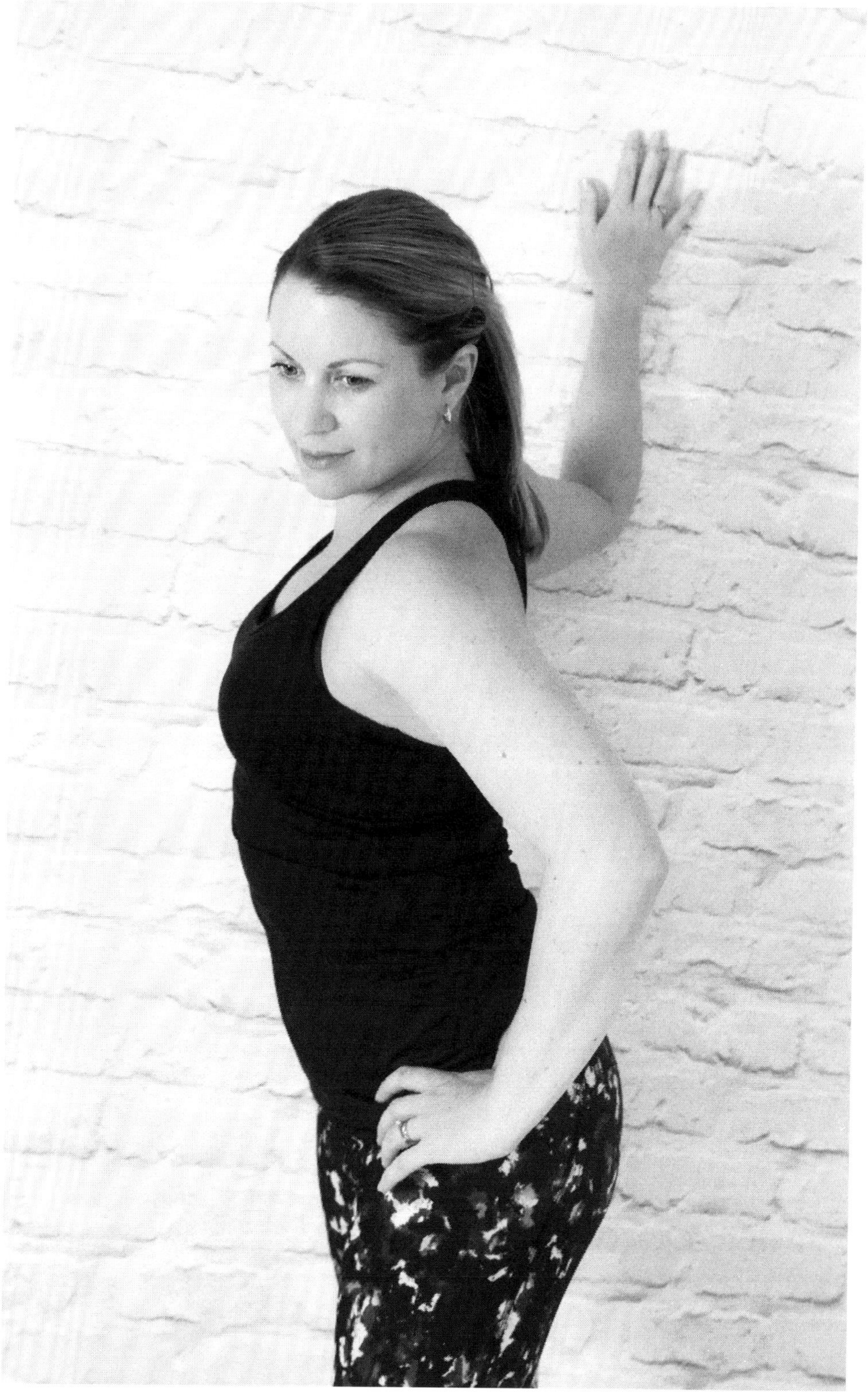

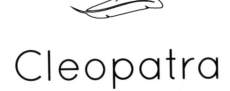

Cleopatra

- Start in your Dumb Waiter position.

- After **inhaling** to open the arms up initially, then **exhale** to stretch the arms out to the sides.

- *Inhale to bring the elbows back into the waist.*

  - **Exhale** to return the hands to the front of the body.

  - Repeat eight times.

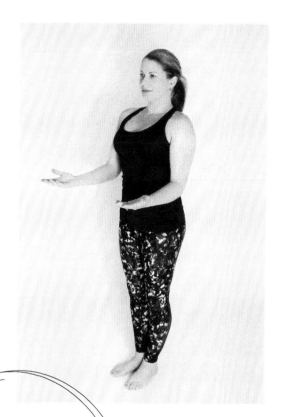

'OPEN
the chest and
keep the back
RELAXED'

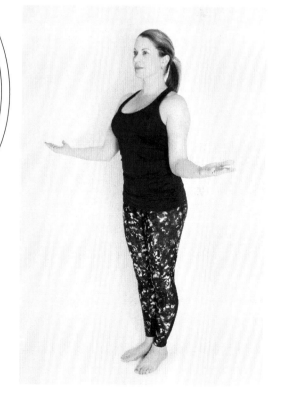

Passing the Water Bottle 1

You might need someone to help you by passing the bottle from hand to hand.

- Stand tall to start, with your water bottle in one hand.

- **Inhale** and take the water bottle over your shoulder and down the back in order to pass it to the other hand, which reaches behind your lower back.

- **Exhale** and swap sides.

- Repeat eight times on each side.

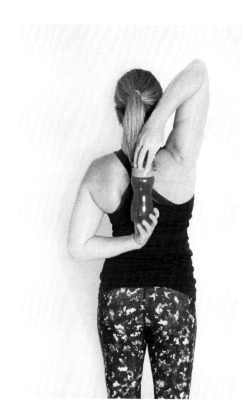

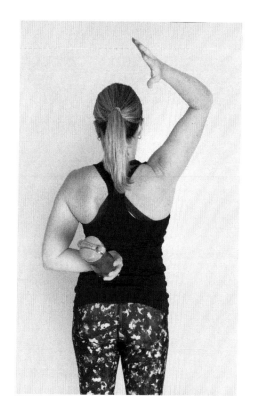

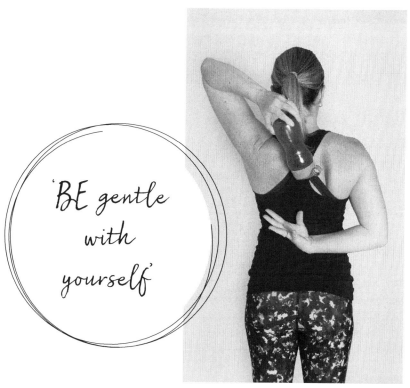

'BE gentle
with
yourself'

Full Single Arm Circles

- Stand tall to start, with one hand on your hip and the other arm out straight in front of you.

- **Inhale** and start to lift the straight arm upwards.

- **Exhale** and circle the arm backwards.

- *Inhale to start again.*

- Repeat eight times in each direction on each side.

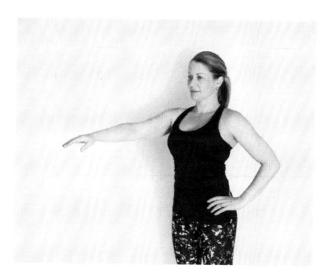

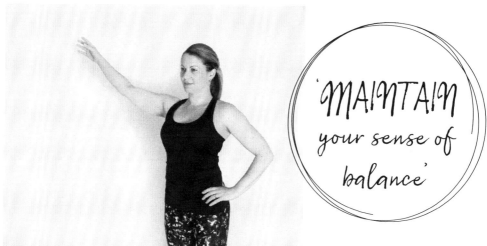

'MAINTAIN your sense of balance'

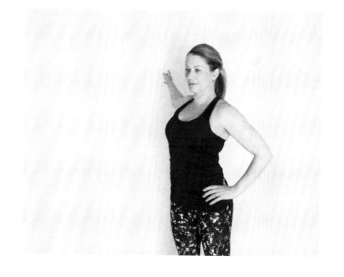

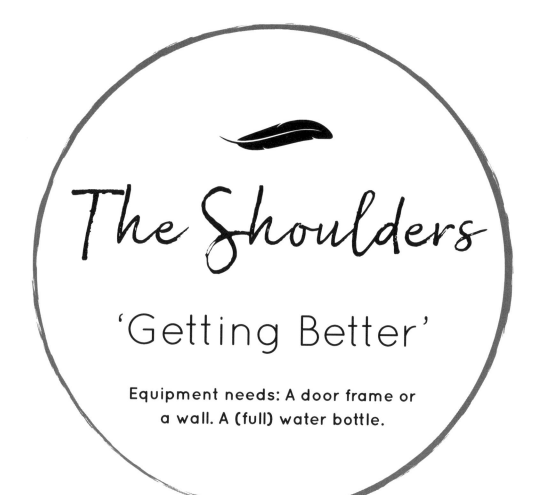

The Shoulders

'Getting Better'

Equipment needs: A door frame or
a wall. A (full) water bottle.

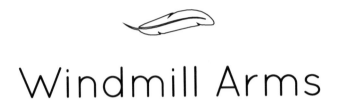

Windmill Arms

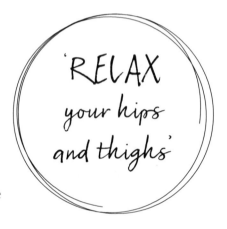

'RELAX your hips and thighs'

- Lie on your back as for Backstroke Arms.

- Place the thin pillow under the back of your head.

- **Inhale** to prepare.

- **Exhale** and take one arm over your head to a point where you can still see your elbow in your peripheral vision.

- **Inhale** to take both arms out to the sides of the body.

- **Exhale** to complete a circular swap over, finishing with the arms vertical.

- **Inhale** and hold the arms in vertical.

- **Exhale** to take the other arm over your head this time.

- Repeat eight times in each direction.

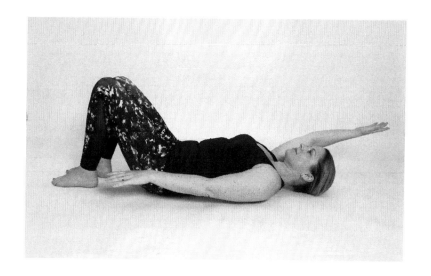

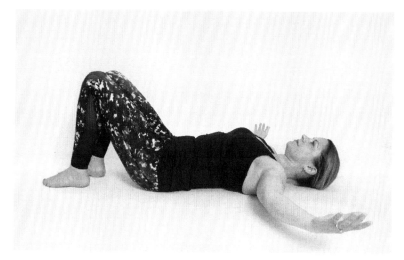

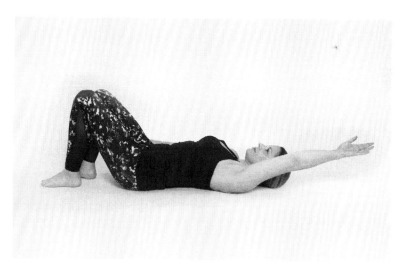

Door Frame/ Wall Stretch 2

- Place one hand on to a wall or against a door frame.

- Keep the arm *straighter*.

- Turn your body away from the arm.

- **Inhale** and **exhale** eight times as you hold the stretch.

- Repeat for eight breath rounds on the other side.

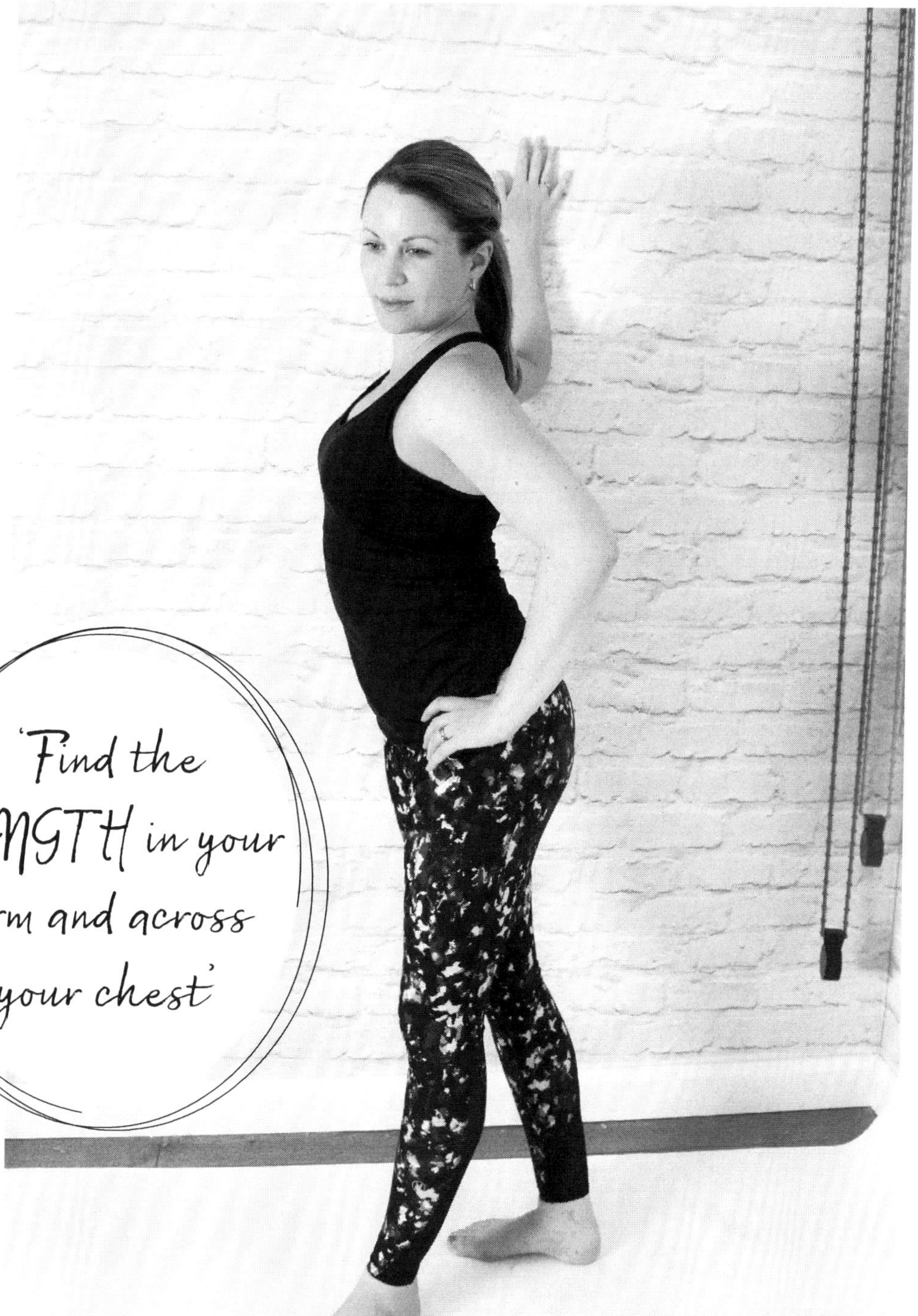

'Find the LENGTH in your arm and across your chest'

Chicken Wings

- Stand tall to start and position the arms as depicted.

- **Inhale** and lengthen the spine.

- **Exhale** to prepare.

- **Inhale** and stretch the arms upwards towards the ceiling (and slightly forwards).

- **Exhale** and draw the elbows back down into the sides of the body.

- *Repeat eight times.*

'FEEL the shoulders relax downwards as you lengthen the spine'

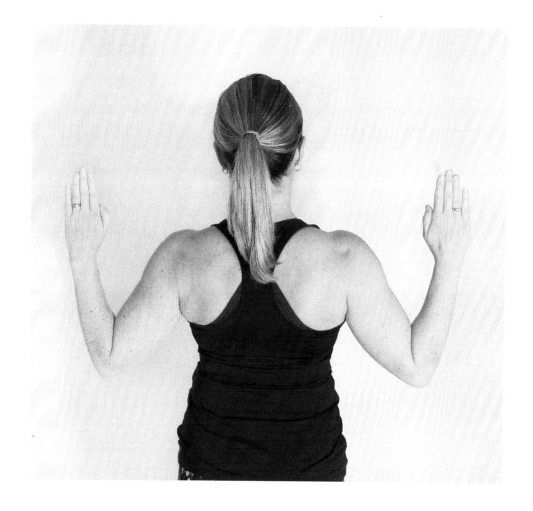

Passing the Water Bottle 2

You should be able to do this now without extra help.

- Stand tall to start, with your water bottle in one hand.

- **Inhale** and take the water bottle over your shoulder and down the back in order to pass it to the other hand, which reaches behind your lower back.

- **Exhale** and swap sides.

- Repeat eight times on each side.

'KEEP the spine straight'

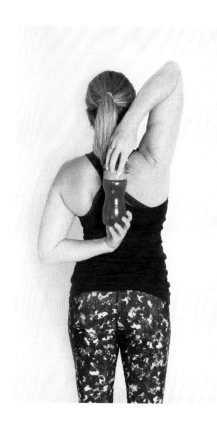
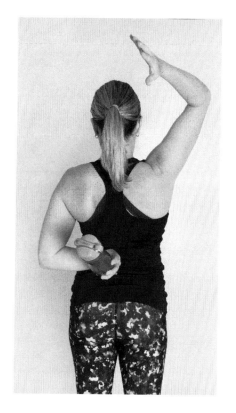

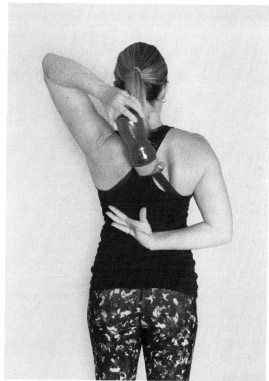

Full Double Arm Circles

- Stand tall to start, with both arms out in front of you.

- **Inhale** and start to lift both arms upwards.

- **Exhale** and circle both arms backwards.

- **Inhale** to start again.

- Repeat eight times in each direction.

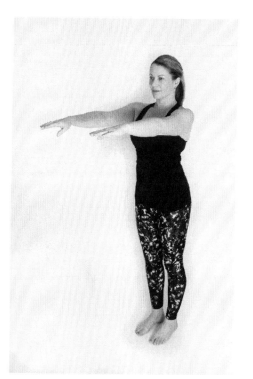

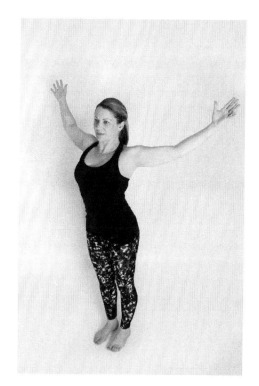

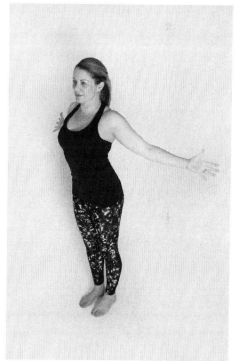

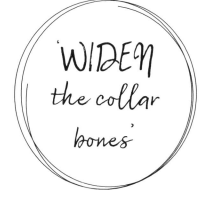

'WIDEN the collar bones'

The Knees

'The Beginning'

Equipment needs: A chair. A thin pillow.

Knee Bends in Standing

- Stand side on to the back of a chair so that you can hold on for support.

- **Inhale** and lengthen through the spine.

- **Exhale** and gently bend both knees.

- **Inhale** to straighten back up.

- Repeat eight times.

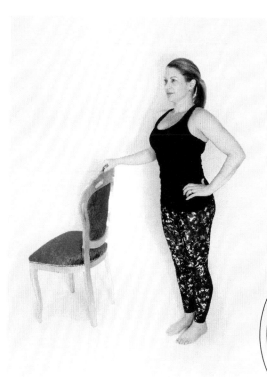

'Maintain the LENGTH in the spine'

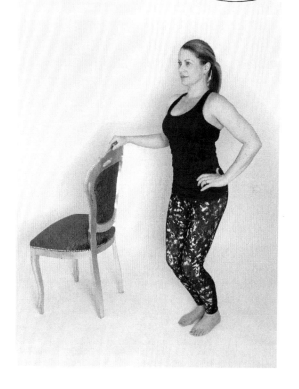

Standing Knee Folds

- Stand side on to the back of a chair so that you can hold on for support.

- **Inhale** and lengthen through the spine.

- **Exhale** and fold one leg up to a 90-degree angle in both the hip and knee.

- **Inhale** to lower back down.

- Repeat eight times on each side.

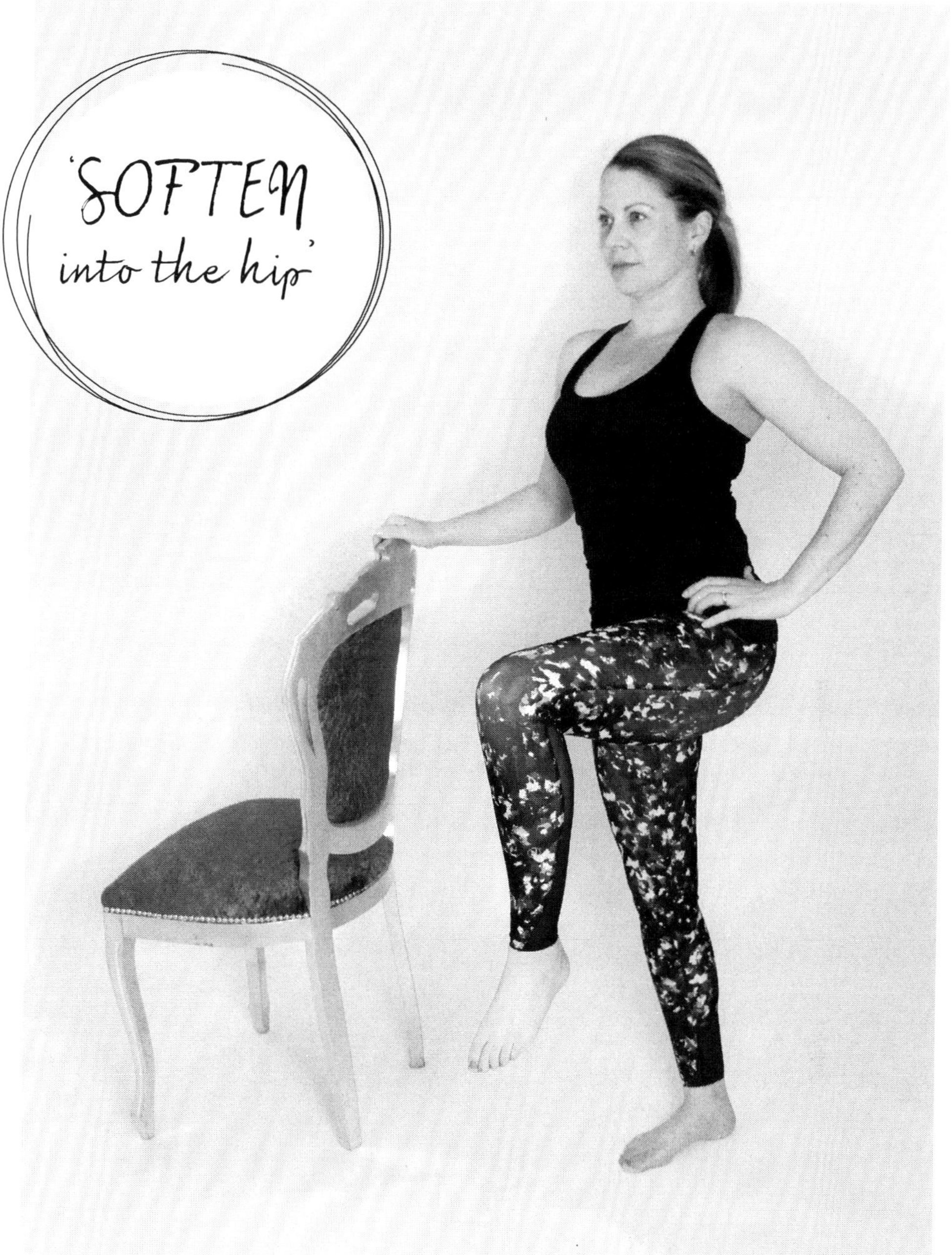
'SOFTEN
into the hip'

Side Lying Knee Bends to Swings

- Lie on your side with your head resting on an outstretched arm (optional to put the thin pillow between the arm and the ear).

- One hand supports firmly, in front of the body.

- Bend the bottom leg and then stretch the top leg out in line with the body.

- **Inhale** to prepare.

- **Exhale** and swing the top leg forwards whilst bending the knee.

- Inhale to take the leg backwards, keeping it straight.

- Repeat eight times on each side.

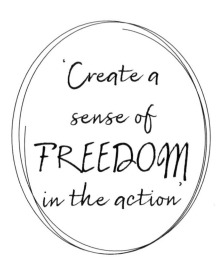

'Create a sense of FREEDOM in the action'

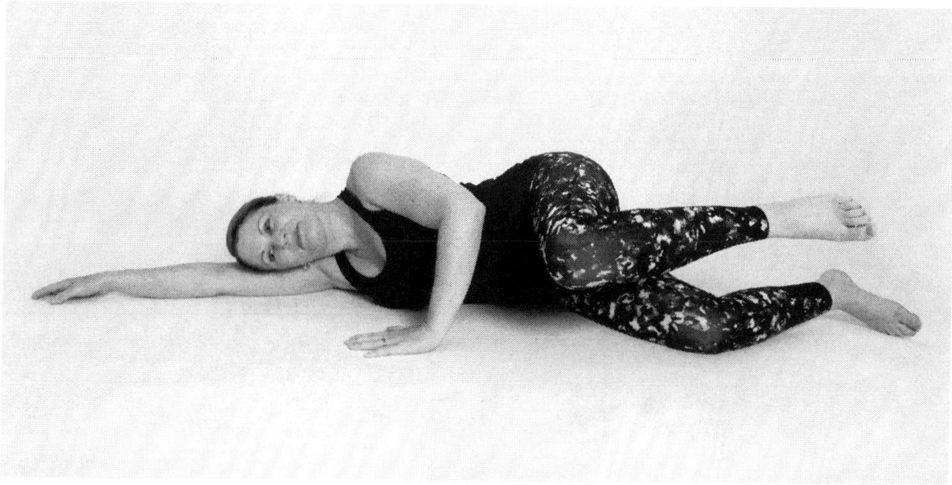

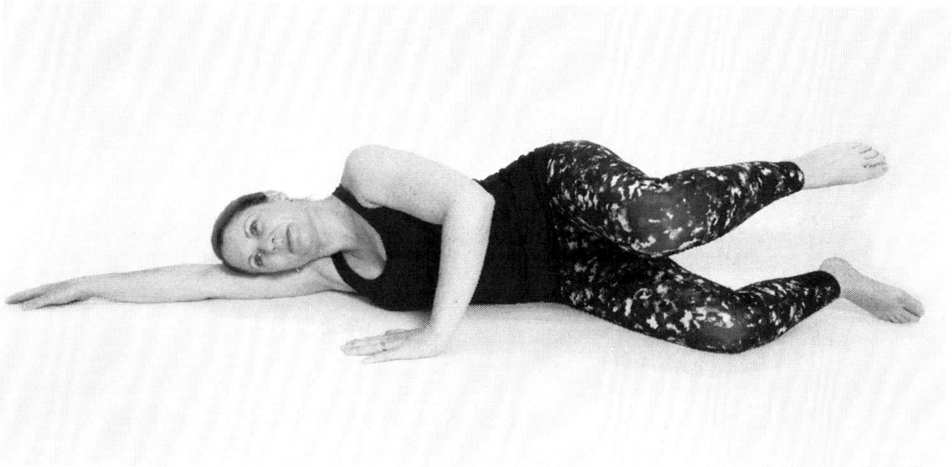

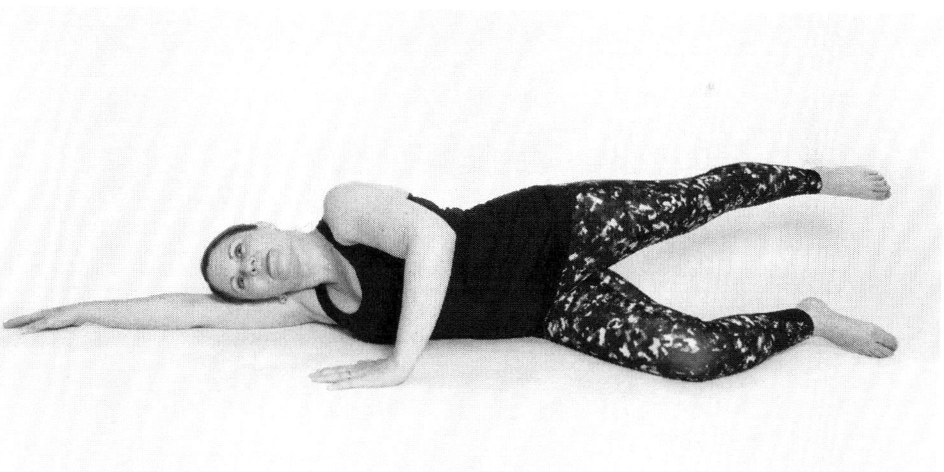

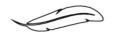

Leg Across Knee Stretch

Also useful for *'The Beginning'* **The Back**

- Lie on your back with your feet hip socket distance apart and on the floor.

- Place the thin pillow under the back of your head.

- Position the outside ankle of one leg on to the thigh of the other leg.

- *You can use your hand to gently push the leg out to the side.*

- **Inhale** and **exhale** for eight breath rounds as you hold the position.

- Repeat on the other side.

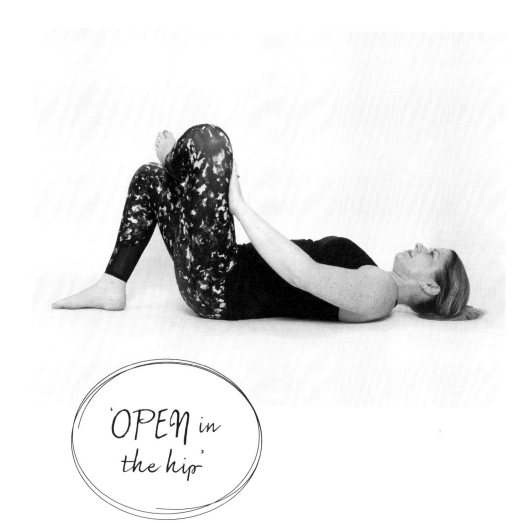

'OPEN in the hip'

Single Straight Leg Raise (on chair)

- Sit tall on your chair.

- **Inhale** and lengthen the spine.

- **Exhale** and straighten one leg lifting it as high as you can.

- **Inhale** to lower back down.

- *Change sides.*

  - Repeat eight times on each side.

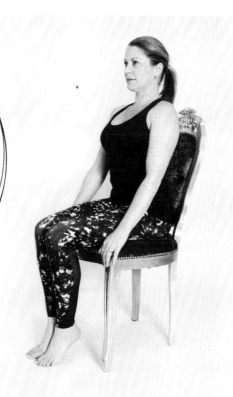

'Maintain the LENGTH in the spine'

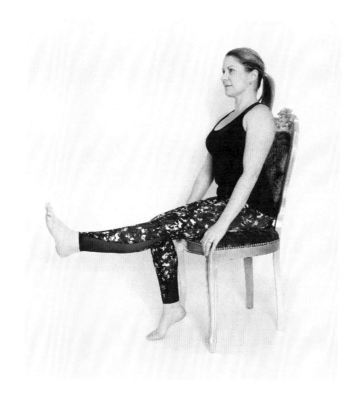

The Knees

'Improving'

Equipment needs: A thin pillow.

Marching Knees

- Stand tall with your hands on your hips.

- **Inhale** and lengthen the spine.

- **Exhale** and bend both knees, lifting one heel at the same time.

- **Inhale** to straighten up.

- Repeat eight times on each side.

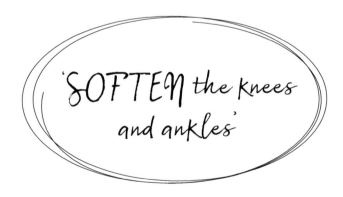

'SOFTEN the knees and ankles'

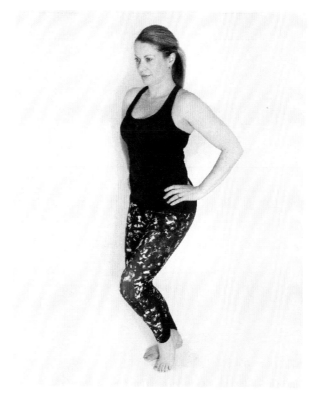

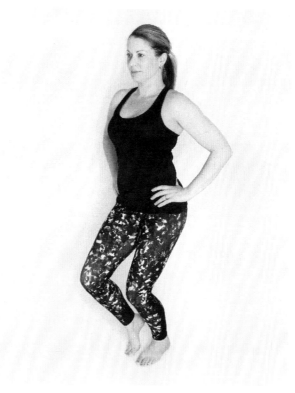

Standing Knee Lifts

- *Stand tall to start.*

  - **Inhale** and lengthen through the spine.

  - **Exhale** and lift one knee up so that you can tap it with one hand.

  - **Inhale** to lower back down.

  - Repeat eight times on each side.

'Focus on maintaining LENGTH in the supporting leg'

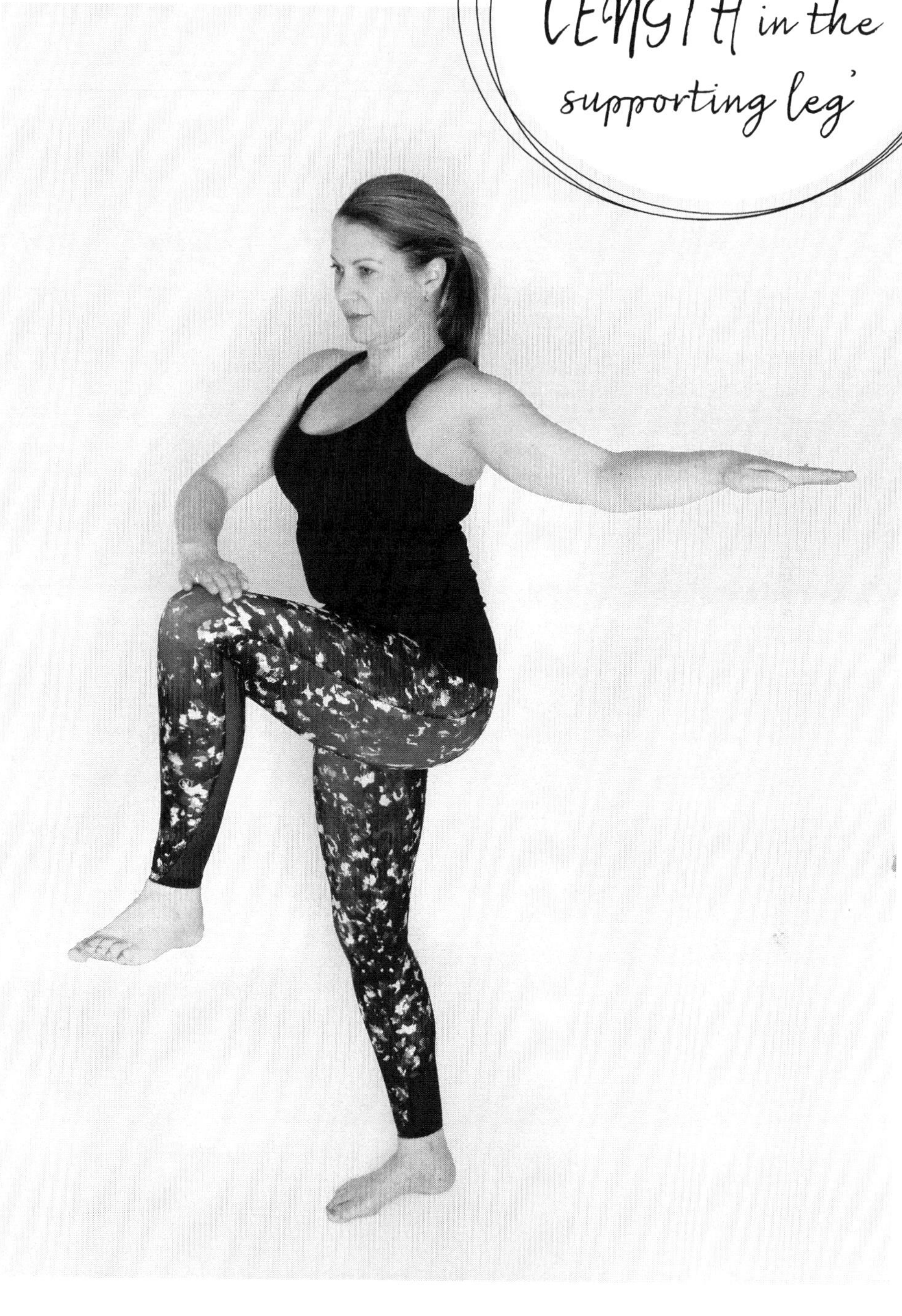

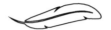

Oyster to Single Leg Extension

- Lie on your side with your head resting on an outstretched arm (optional to put the thin pillow between the arm and the ear).

- One hand supports firmly, in front of the body.

- Line the feet up with the spine, knees bent.

- *Feet need to be slightly off the floor, knees down.*

- **Inhale** to prepare.

- **Exhale** and keep the feet together as you lift open the top knee.

- *Use the supporting hand to help push the knee a little further out if possible.*

- **Inhale** and then stretch the top leg out in front of you.

- **Exhale** to bend it back to Oyster.

- **Inhale** to close the knees.

- Repeat eight times on each side.

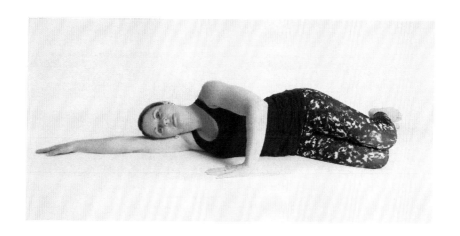

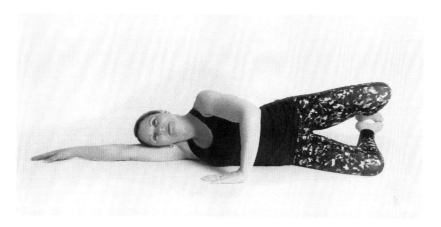

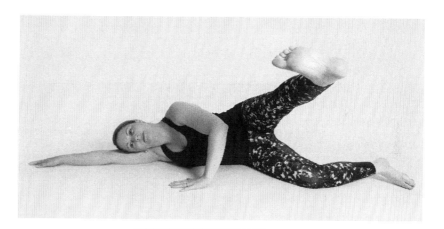

'Maintain the LENGTH through your waist'

Figure of 4 Stretch 1

Also useful for *'Improving'* **The Back**

- Lie on your back with your feet hip socket distance apart and on the floor.

- Place the thin pillow under the back of your head.

- Position the outside ankle of one leg on to the thigh of the other leg.

- Now lift up the leg that was still on the floor and hold round the back of that thigh.

- **Inhale** and **exhale** for eight breath rounds as you hold the position.

- Repeat on the other side.

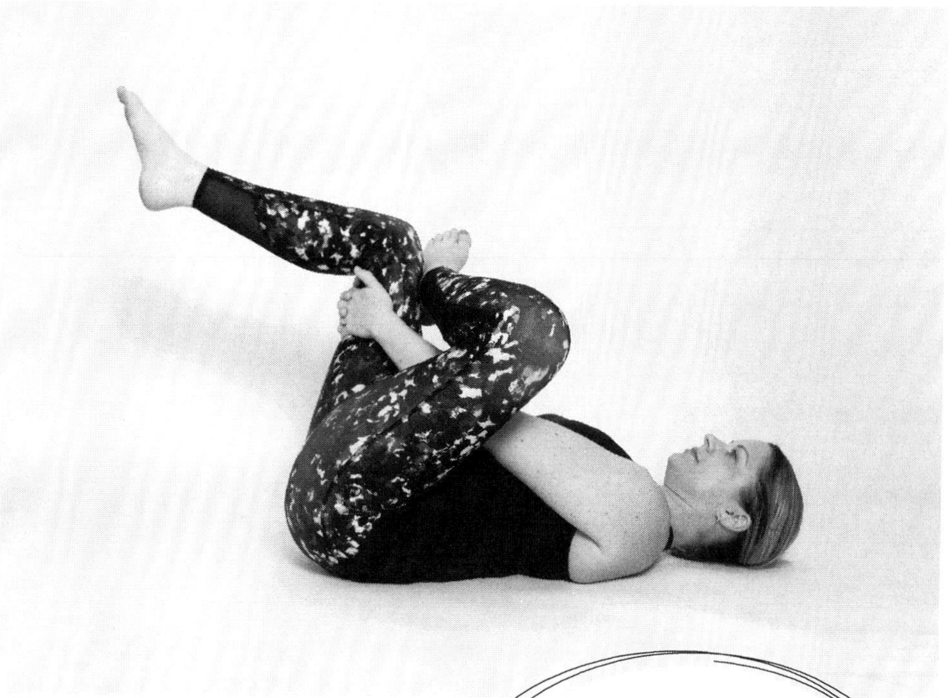

'RELAX your shoulders'

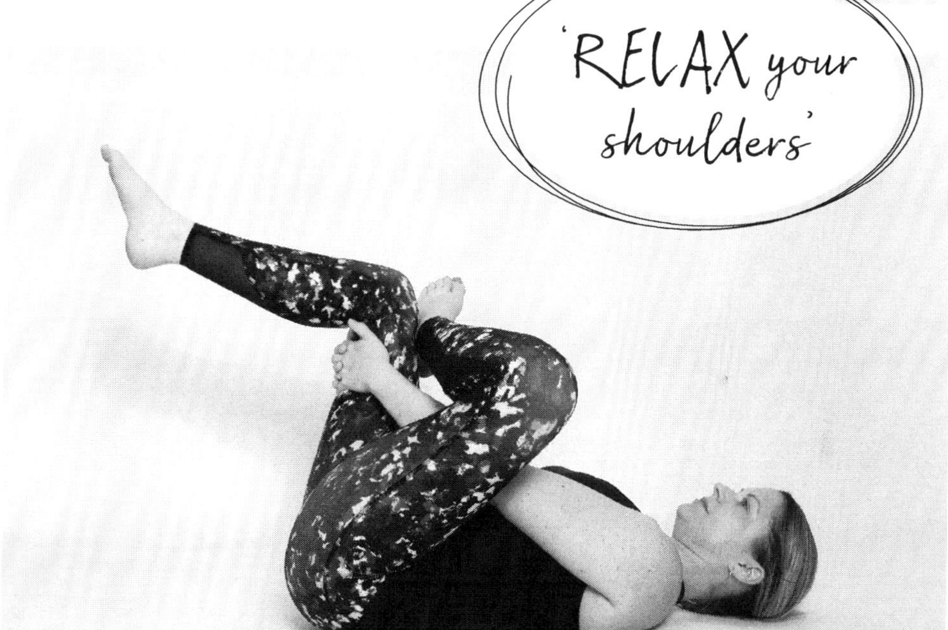

Supine Straight Single Leg Raise 1

- Lie on your back with the thin pillow under your head.

- *One leg will stay bent, foot flat.*

  - Stretch the other leg up towards the ceiling.

  - **Inhale** to prepare.

  - **Exhale** to lower the straight leg down towards the floor.

  - **Inhale** to lift it back up.

  - Repeat eight times on each side.

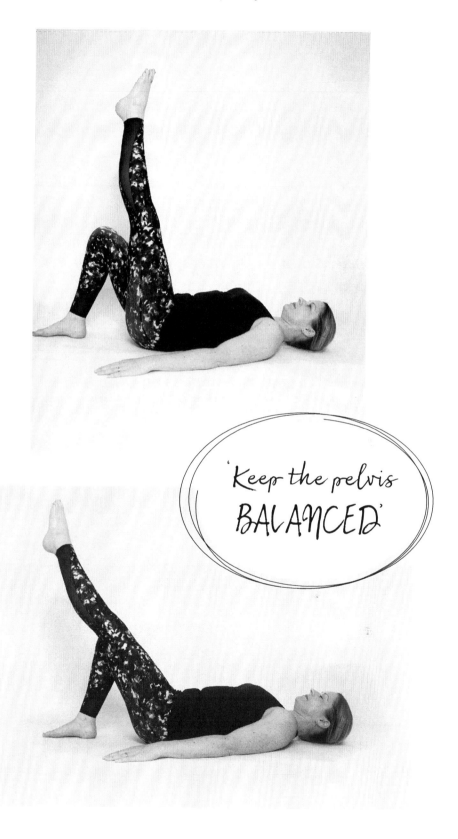

'Keep the pelvis
BALANCED'

The Knees

'Getting Better'

Equipment needs: A thin pillow.

Deep Marching Knees

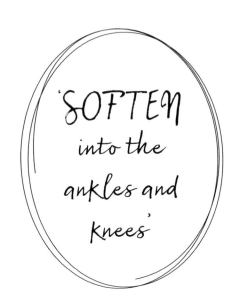

'SOFTEN into the ankles and knees'

- Stand tall with your hands on your hips.

- **Inhale** and lengthen the spine.

- **Exhale** and bend both knees, lifting one heel at the same time as leaning forwards from the waist.

- **Inhale** to straighten up and then rise up on to the toes.

- Repeat eight times on each side.

1

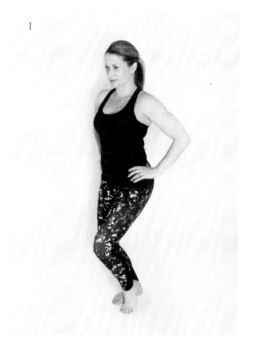

2

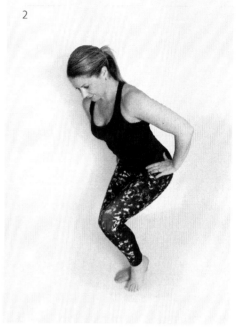

3

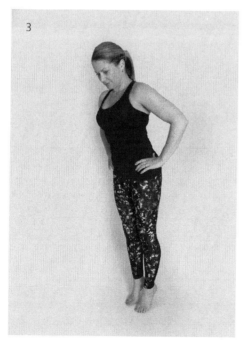

4

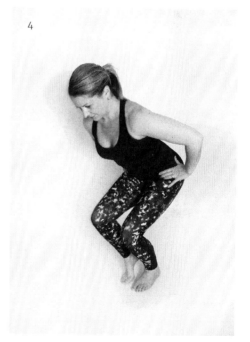

Knee Pull Ins

- Stand tall to start.

- **Inhale** and lengthen through the spine.

- **Exhale** and lift one knee up so that you can grab on to it and draw it tightly in towards the body.

- **Inhale** and hold.

- **Exhale** to lower back to the floor.

- Repeat eight times on each side.

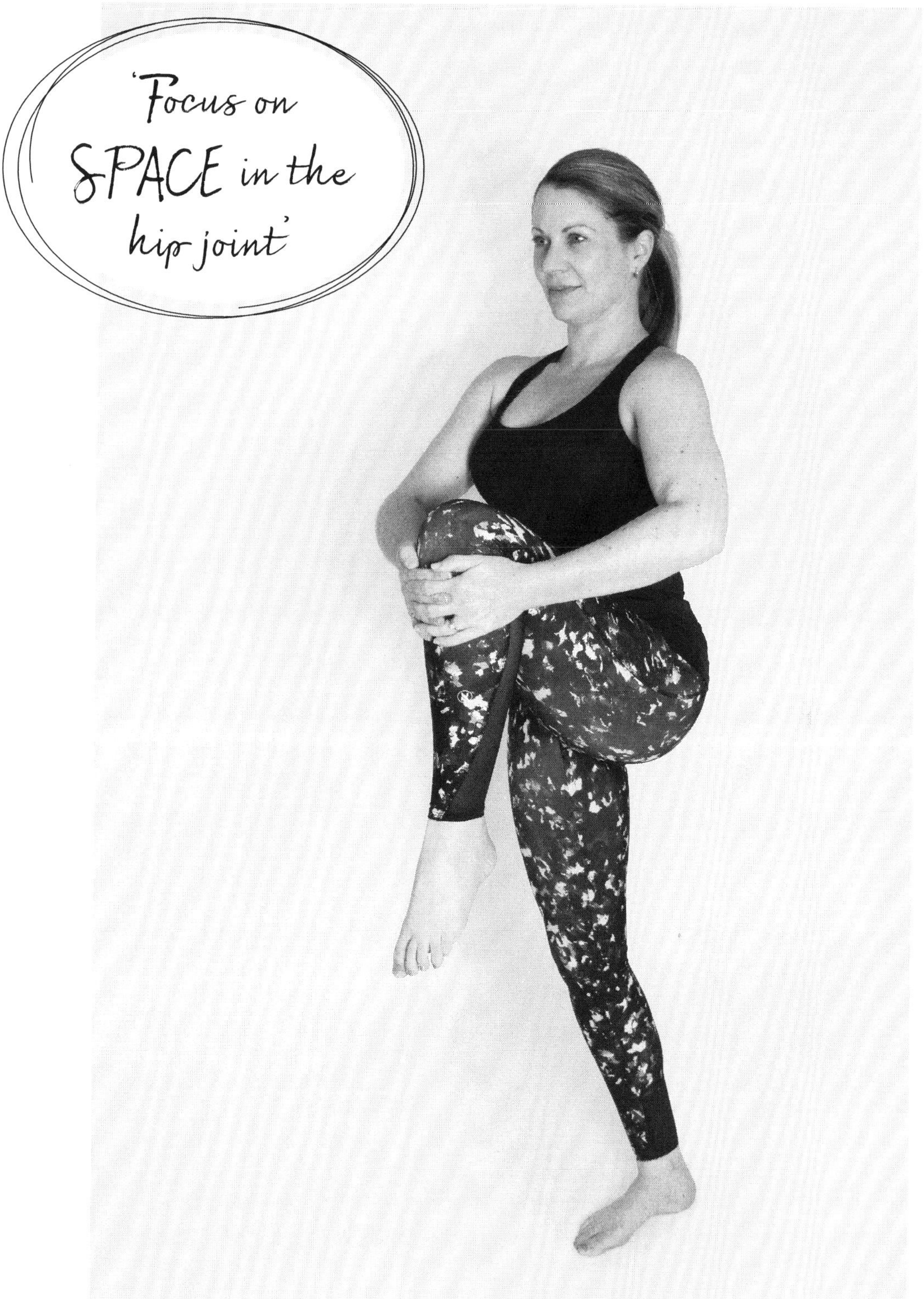
'Focus on
SPACE in the
hip joint'

Oyster to Double Leg Extension

- Lie on your side with your head resting on an outstretched arm (optional to put the thin pillow between the arm and the ear).

- One hand supports firmly, in front of the body.

- Line the feet up with the spine, knees bent.

- *Feet need to be slightly off the floor, knees down.*

- **Inhale** to prepare.

- **Exhale** and keep the feet together as you lift open the top knee.

- *Use the supporting hand to help push the knee a little further out if possible.*

- **Inhale** and then stretch both the legs out in front of you.

- **Exhale** to bend both legs back to Oyster.

- **Inhale** to close the knees.

- Repeat eight times on each side.

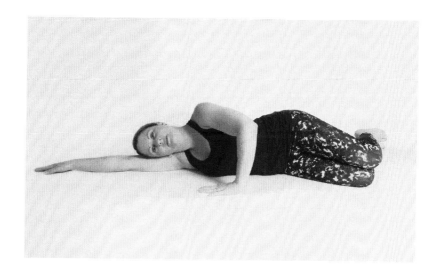

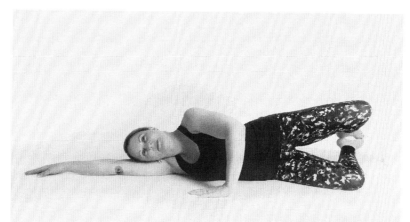

'Try and keep the knees in place when STRETCHING out'

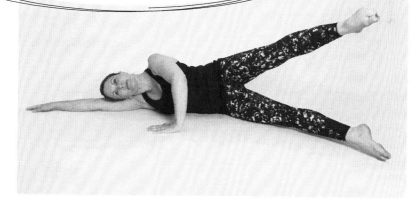

Figure of 4 Stretch 2

Also useful for *'Getting Better'* **The Back**

- Lie on your back with your feet hip socket distance apart and on the floor.

- Place the thin pillow under the back of your head.

- Position the outside ankle of one leg on to the thigh of the other leg.

- Now lift up the leg that was still on the floor and hold on to the front of that shin.

- **Inhale** and **exhale** for eight breath rounds as you hold the position.

- Repeat on the other side.

'RELAX your shoulders'

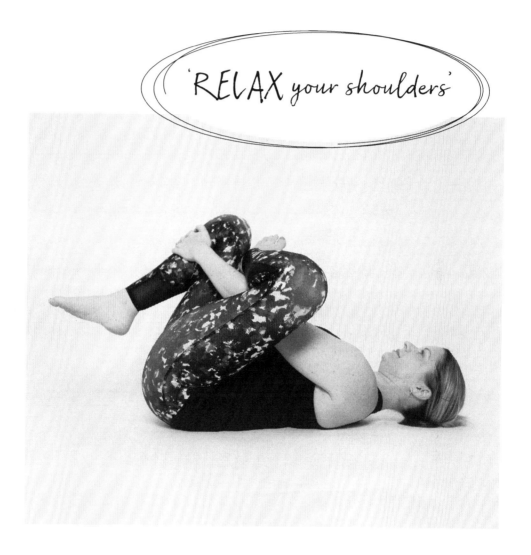

Supine Straight Single Leg Raise 2

- Lie on your back with the thin pillow under your head.

- Stretch one leg out along the floor and slightly out to the side.

- Stretch the other leg up towards the ceiling.

- **Inhale** to prepare.

- **Exhale** to lower the straight leg down towards the floor.

- **Inhale** to lift it back up.

- Repeat eight times on each side.

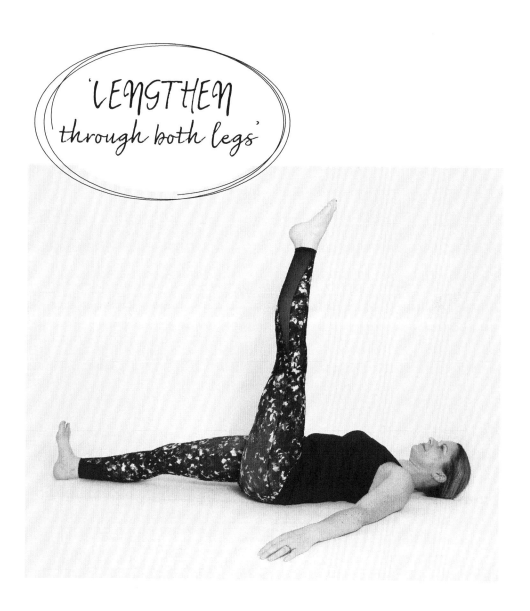

'LENGTHEN
through both legs'

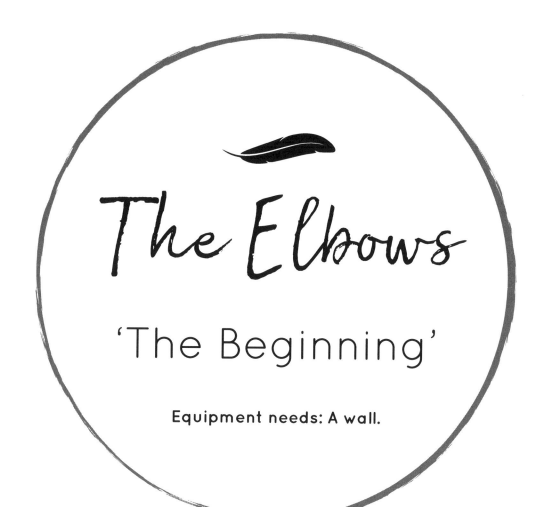

The Elbows

'The Beginning'

Equipment needs: A wall.

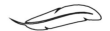

Wrist Down/Wrist Up

Also useful for *'The Beginning'* **The Wrists and Hands**

- Either sit or stand in a comfortable position.

- Hold one arm out in front of you.

- **Inhale** and turn the palm up, allow the action to travel through the arm to the shoulder.

- **Exhale** and turn the palm down.

- Repeat for eight breaths on each side.

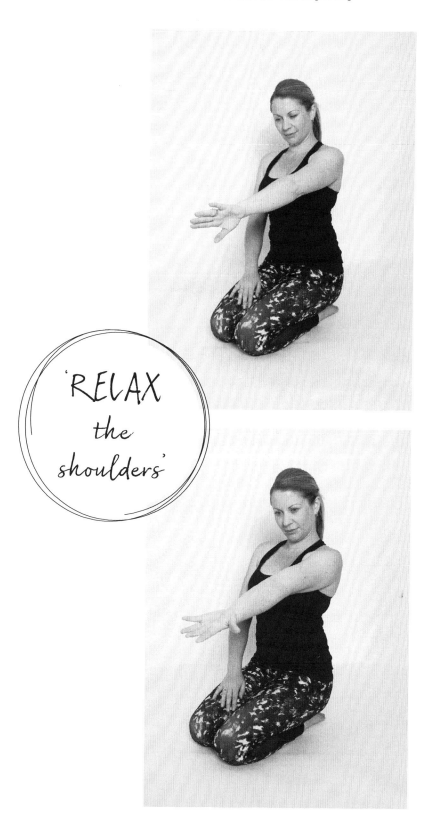

'RELAX the shoulders'

'Weightless' Bicep Curls

- From the same starting position as for Wrist Down/Wrist Up.

- Make a fist.

- **Inhale** to prepare.

- **Exhale** to curl the fist in towards your shoulder.

- **Inhale** to stretch away.

- Repeat eight times on each arm.

'FEEL the length through the back of the upper arm'

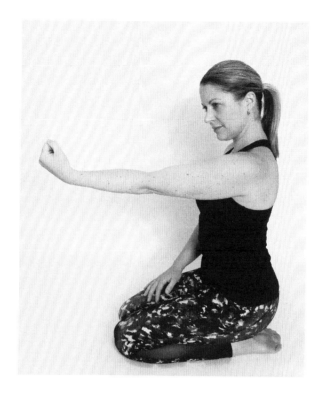

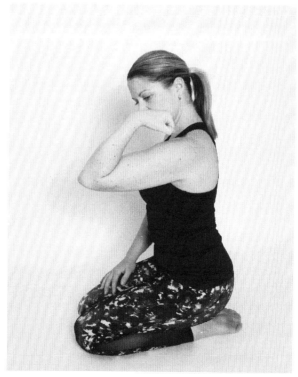

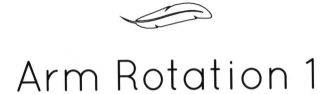

Arm Rotation 1

- Stand facing a wall and place the back of your hand against it.

- **Inhale** and turn your elbow outwards without moving the hand.

- **Exhale** and turn the elbow crease to face the ceiling.

- Repeat for eight breaths on each side.

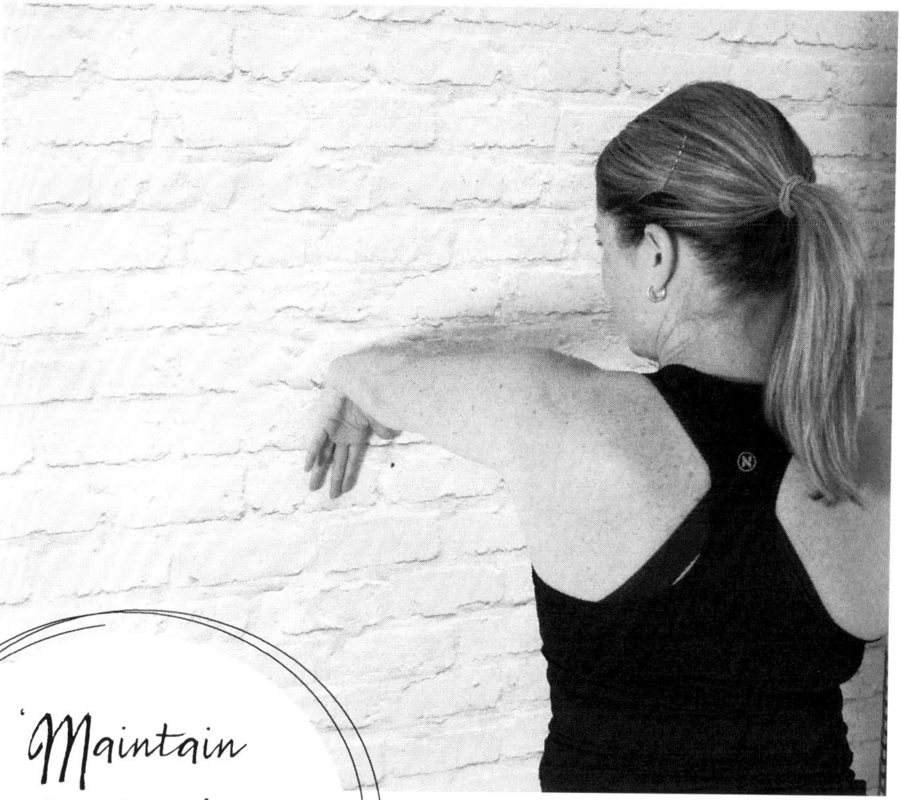

'Maintain LENGTH in the spine'

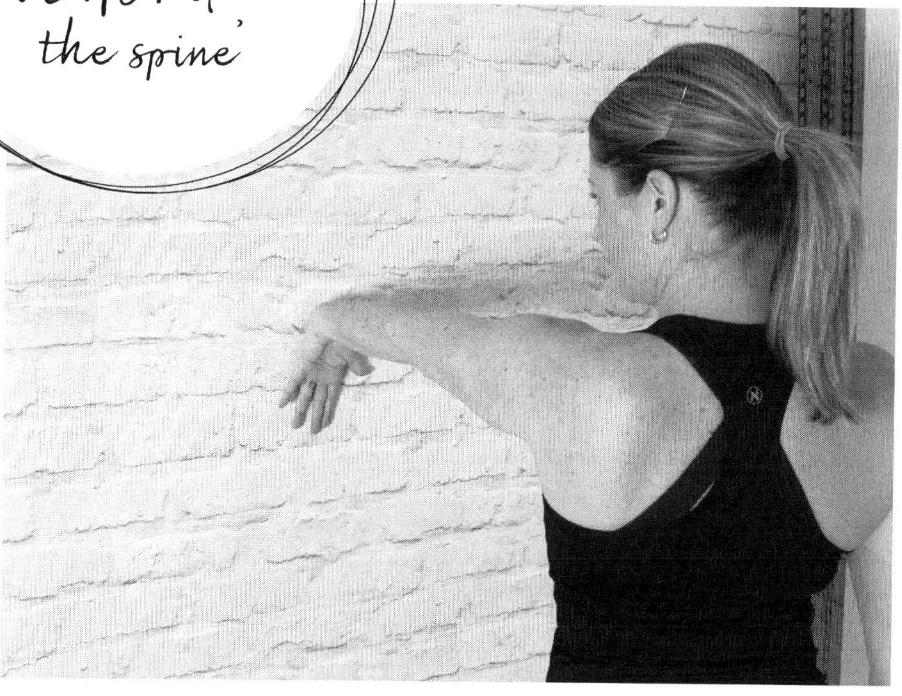

Hanging/Turning Arms

Also useful for *'The Beginning'* **The Shoulders**

- Either sit or stand in a comfortable position.

- Hold one arm down by your side.

- **Inhale** and turn the palm up, allow the action to travel through the arm to the shoulder.

- **Exhale** and turn the palm round the other way.

- Repeat for eight breaths on each side.

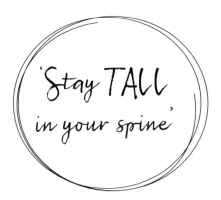

'Stay TALL in your spine'

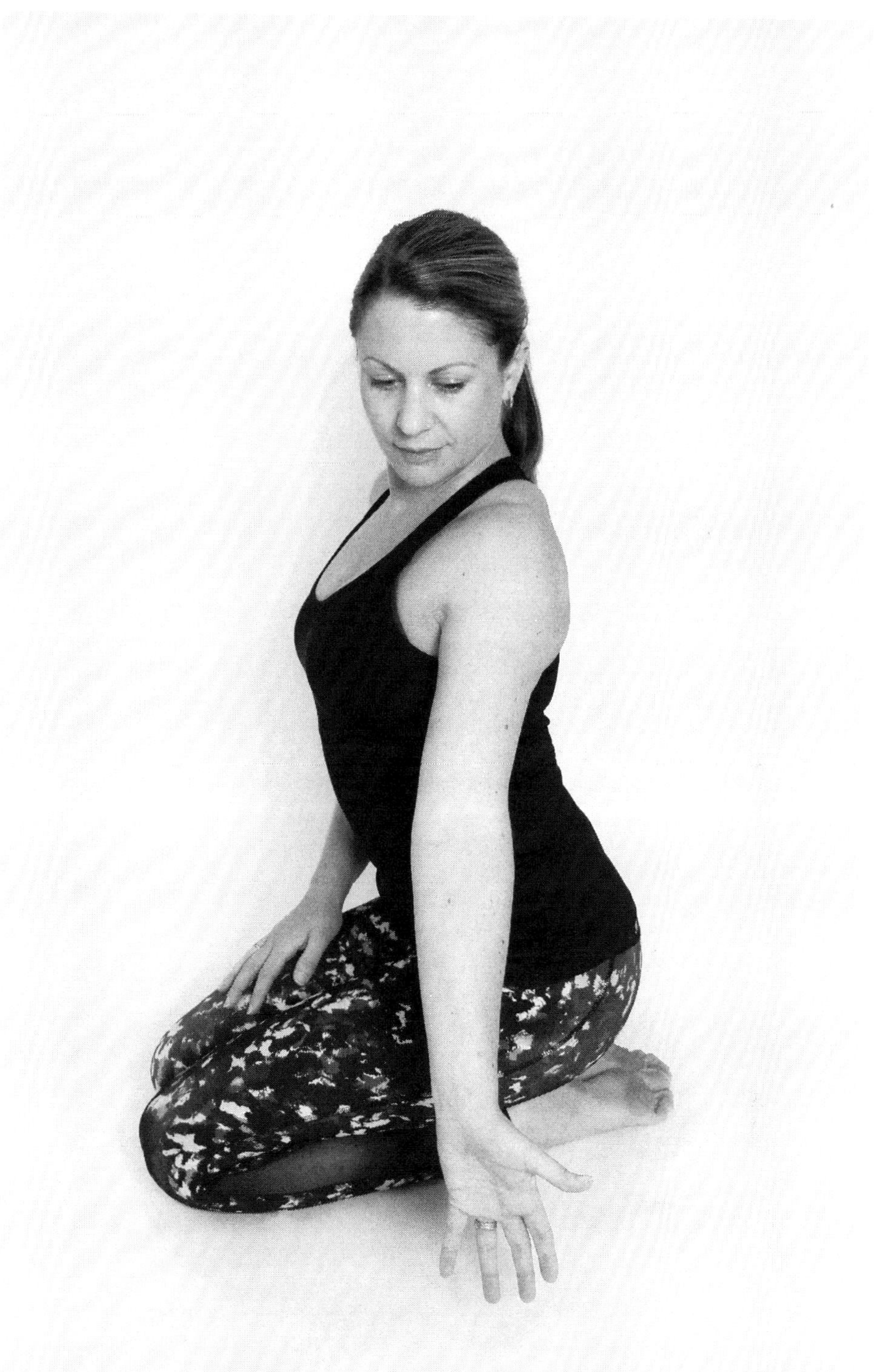

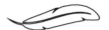

Lower Arm Circles

- Either sit or stand in a comfortable position.

- Hold one arm down by your side.

  - **Inhale** and circle the lower arm in one direction.

  - **Exhale** and circle the arm again in the same direction.

  - Repeat for eight breaths in each direction.

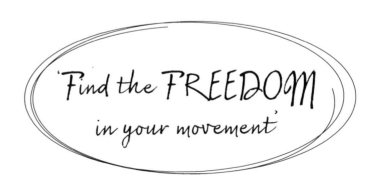

'Find the FREEDOM in your movement'

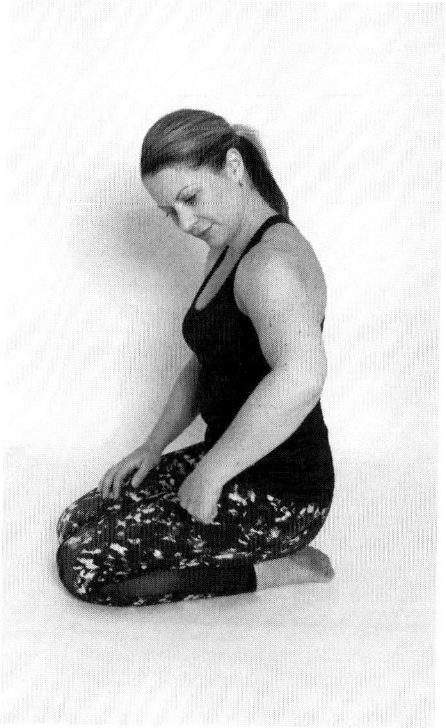

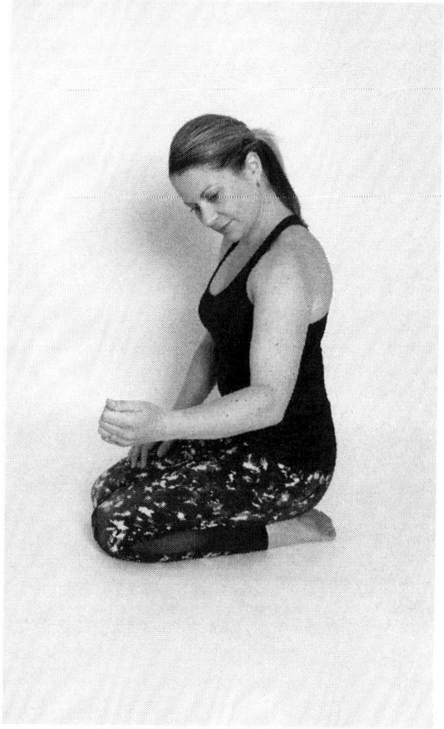

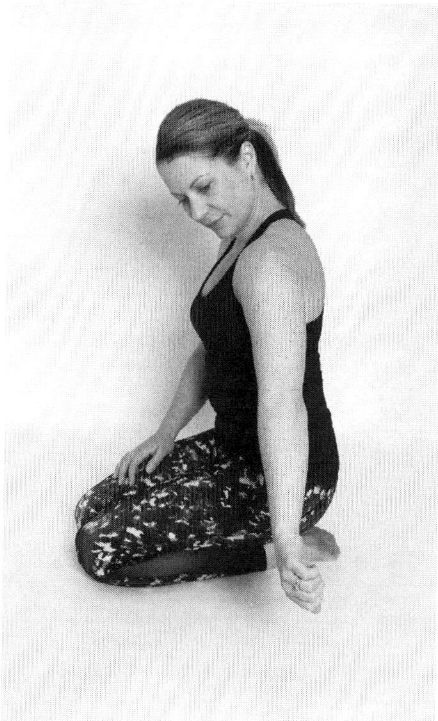

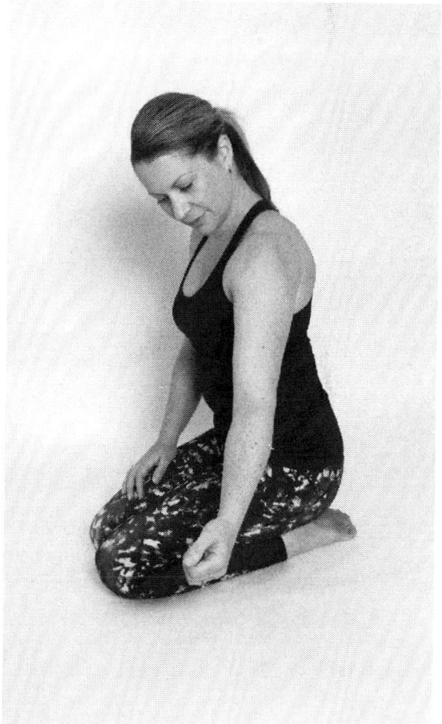

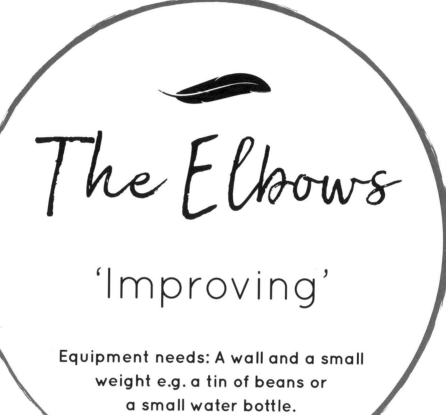

The Elbows

'Improving'

Equipment needs: A wall and a small
weight e.g. a tin of beans or
a small water bottle.

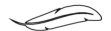

Weighted Wrist Up/ Wrist Down

Also useful for *'Improving'* **The Wrists and Hands**

- Either sit or stand in a comfortable position.

- Hold one arm out in front of you with your weight.

- **Inhale** and turn the palm up, allow the action to travel through the arm to the shoulder.

- **Exhale** and turn the palm down.

- Repeat for eight breaths on each side.

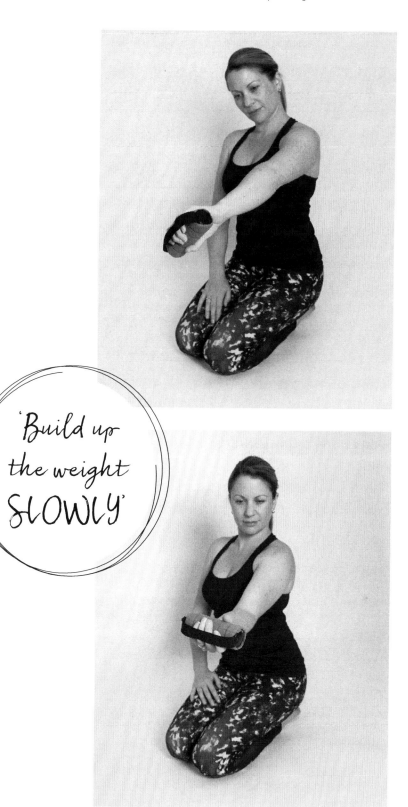

'Build up
the weight
SLOWLY'

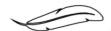

'Weighted' Bicep Curls

From the same starting position as for 'Weightless' Bicep Curls:

- Hold the weight in your hand.

- **Exhale** to curl the weight in towards your shoulder.

- **Inhale** to stretch away.

- Repeat eight times on each arm.

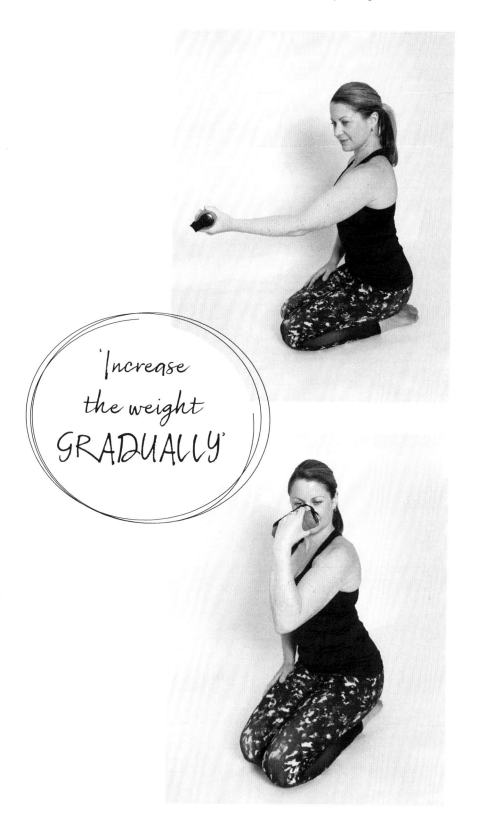

'Increase
the weight
GRADUALLY'

Arm Rotation 2

- Stand facing a wall as for Arm Rotation 1.

- *Place the back of your hand against the wall.*

  - **Inhale** and turn your elbow outwards without moving the hand.

  - **Exhale** and turn the elbow crease to face the ceiling.

  - Repeat for eight breaths on each side

  - Then place your palm against the wall and repeat the above actions.

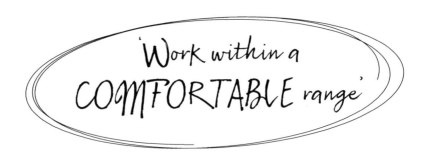

'Work within a COMFORTABLE range'

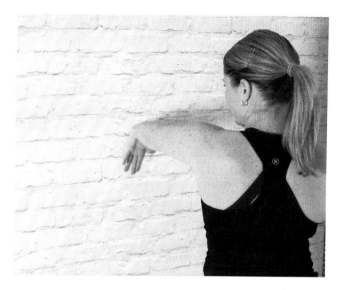

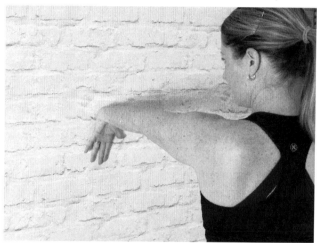

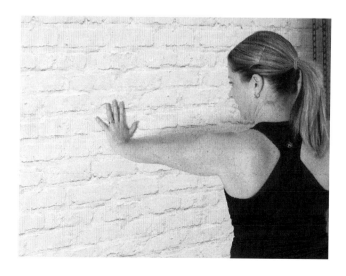

Arm Across Chest

Also useful for *'Improving'* **The Shoulders**

- Either sit or stand in a comfortable position.

- **Inhale** and take your arm out to the side.

- **Exhale** and take the arm across your chest, use your free arm to gently draw the leg across further.

- Hold the stretch for eight breaths.

- Repeat on the other side.

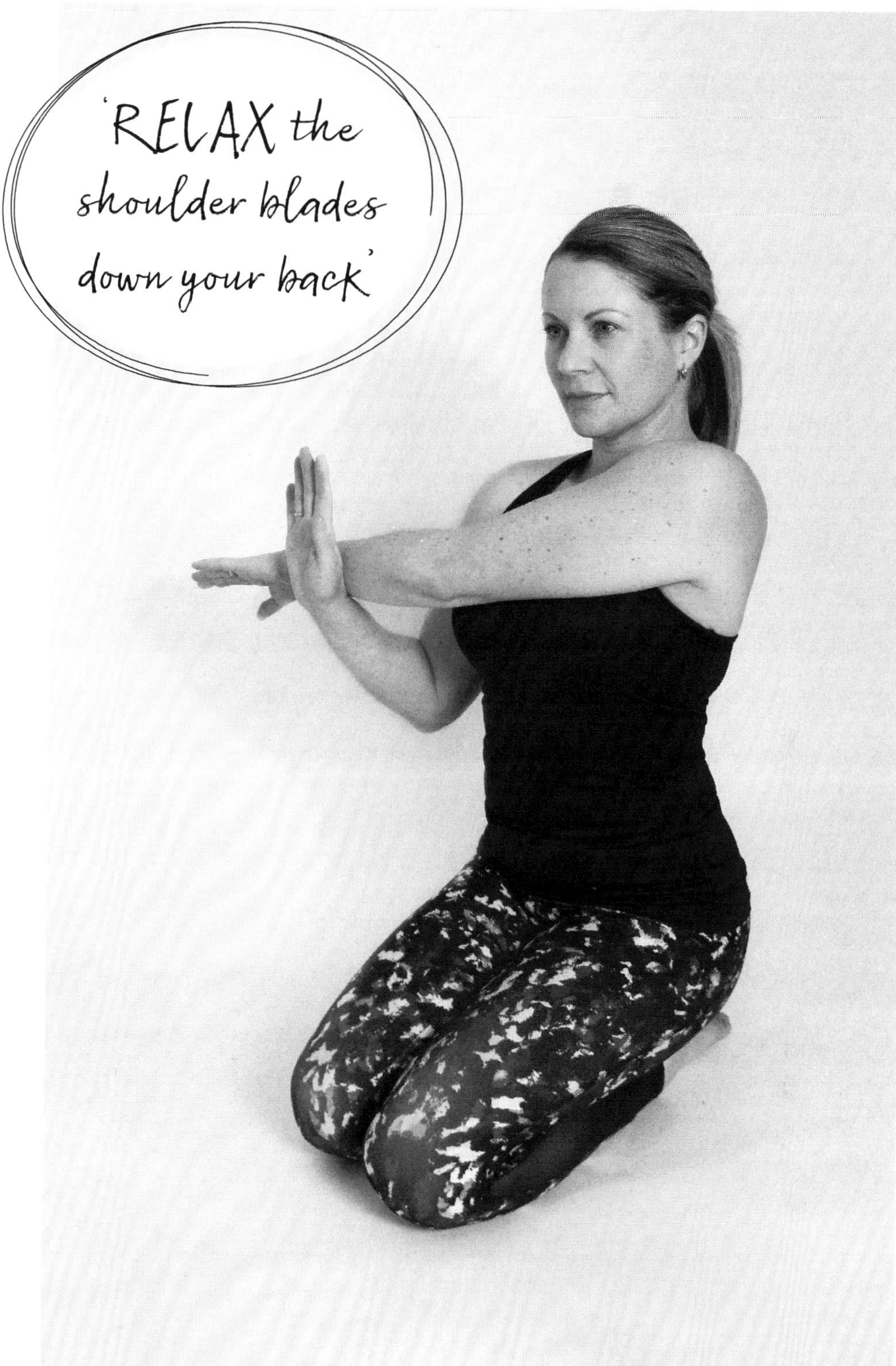
'RELAX the shoulder blades down your back'

Triceps Stretch

Also useful for *'Getting Better'* **The Shoulders**

- Either sit or stand in a comfortable position.

- **Inhale** and take your arm over your shoulder and behind your back.

- **Exhale** and gently press your other hand against the upper arm.

- *Hold the stretch for eight breaths.*

- Repeat on the other side.

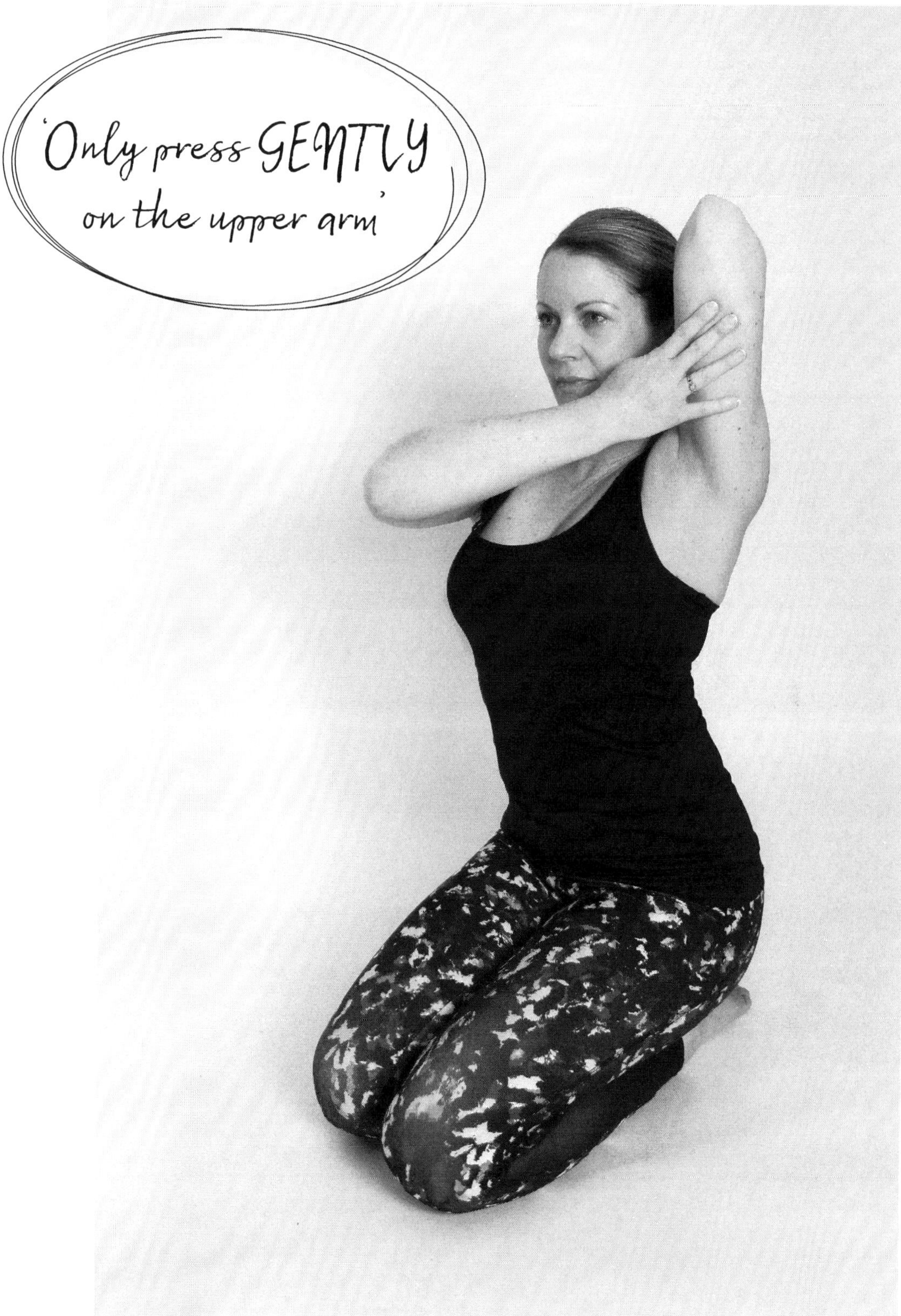
'Only press GENTLY on the upper arm'

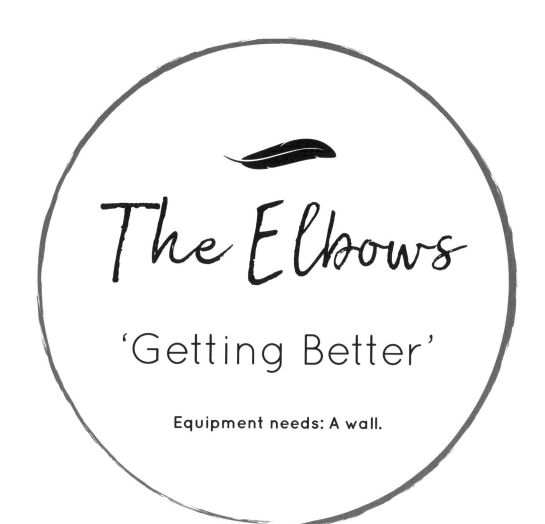

The Elbows

'Getting Better'

Equipment needs: A wall.

'Lizard' on Sand

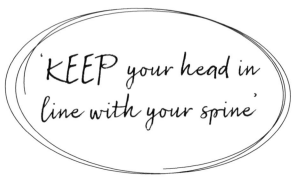

'KEEP your head in line with your spine'

- Start on all fours, hands underneath the shoulders and knees underneath the hips.

- Allow the natural curves in your spine to sit comfortably.

- **Inhale** to prepare.

- **Exhale** and slowly peel one hand away from the floor, bending the elbow and replace it.

- Repeat eight times on each side.

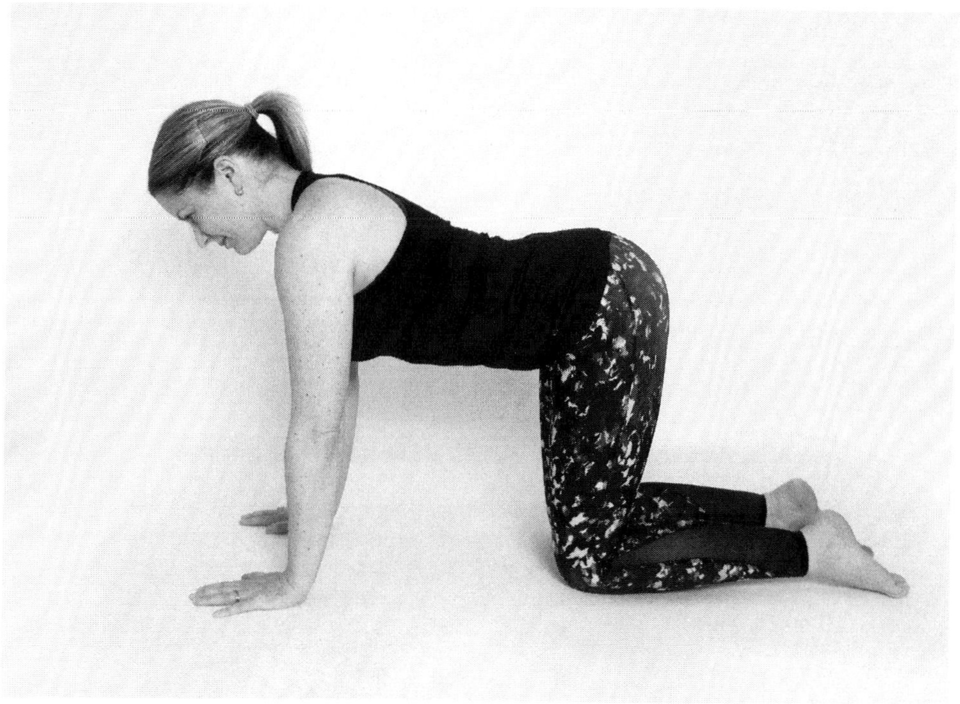

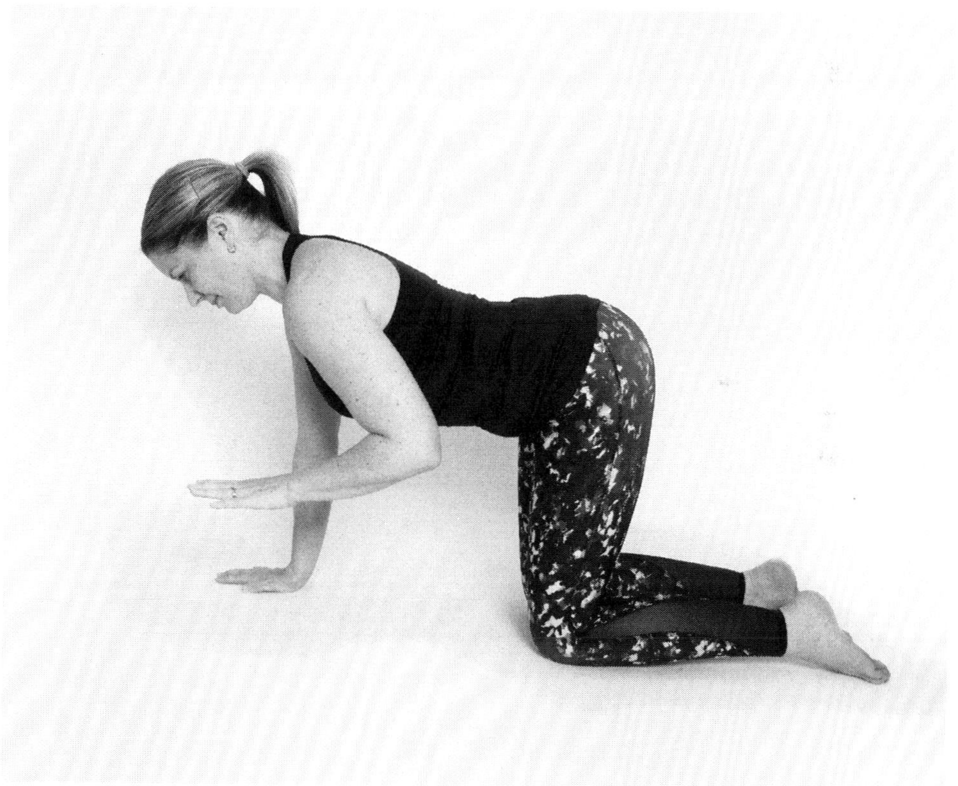

Mini Press Up Against Wall

- Stand facing the wall with your hands shoulder distance apart, palms flat.

- **Inhale** to prepare.

- **Exhale** and bend both elbows, leaning your chest in between your hands and return to the start.

- Repeat eight times.

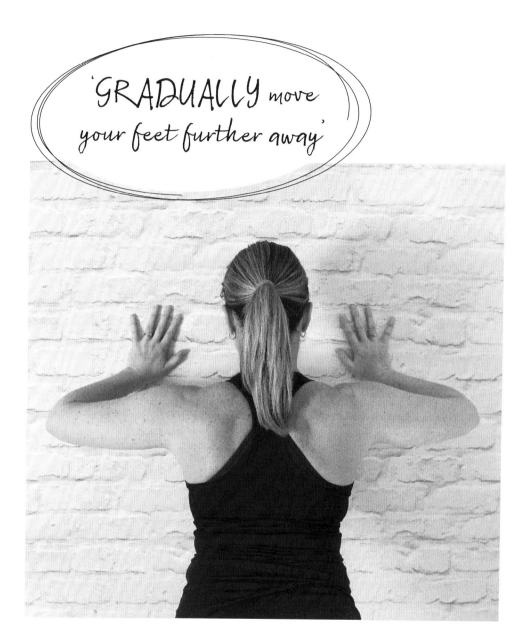

'GRADUALLY move your feet further away'

Arms Stretch Forward

- Either sit or stand in a comfortable position.

- **Inhale** and take both your arms out in front of you, lace the fingers together.

- **Exhale** and push the backs of the hands away from you whilst rounding through the upper back.

- Hold the stretch for eight breaths.

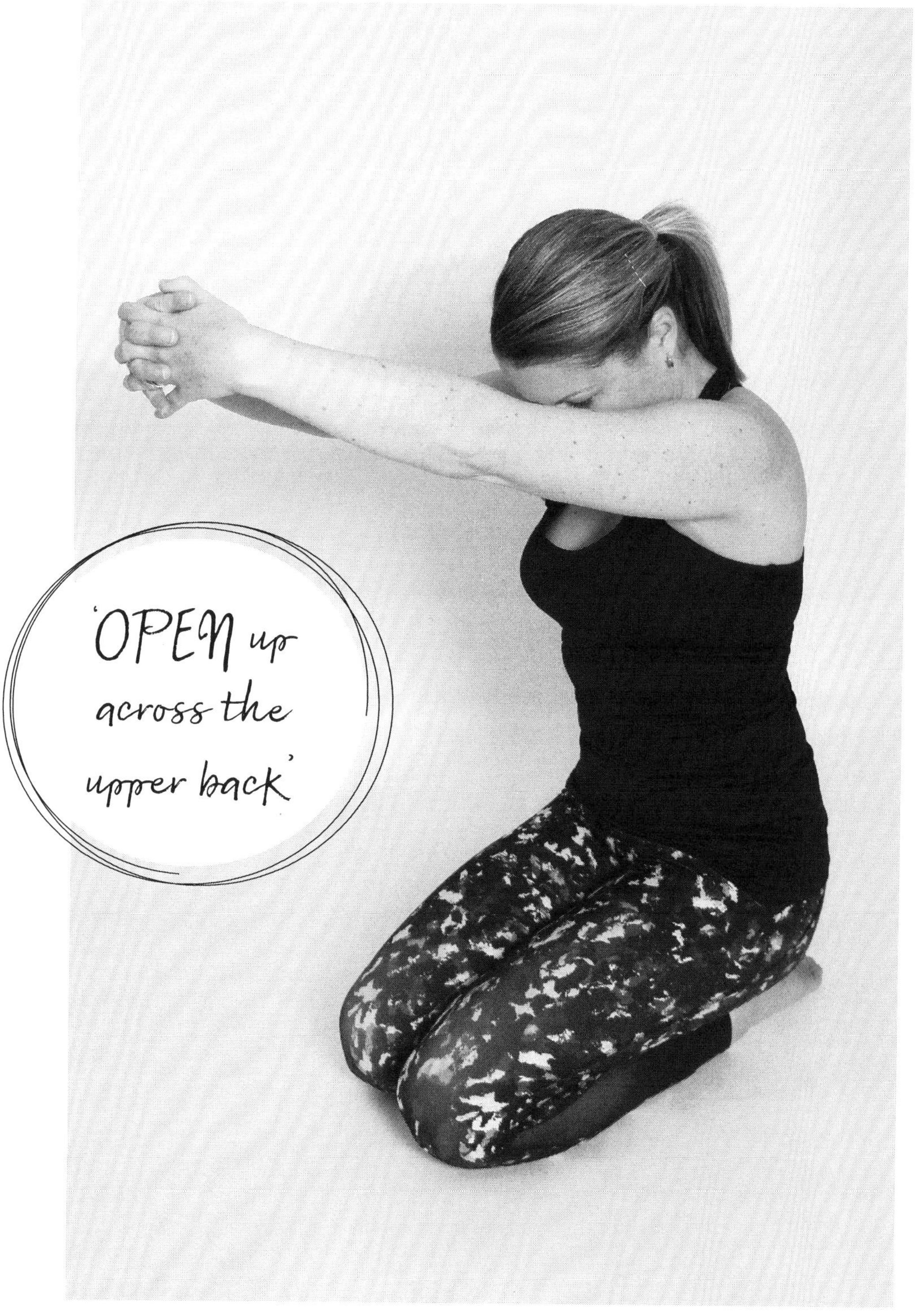
'OPEN up
across the
upper back'

Cow's Face Pose (Arms)

- Either sit or stand in a comfortable position.

- **Inhale** and take one arm over your shoulder and down your back.

- **Exhale** and reach the other arm around your lower back to try and lace the fingers together.

- Hold the stretch for eight breaths.

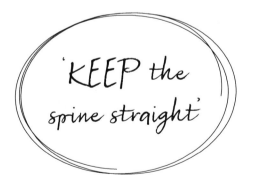

'KEEP the spine straight'

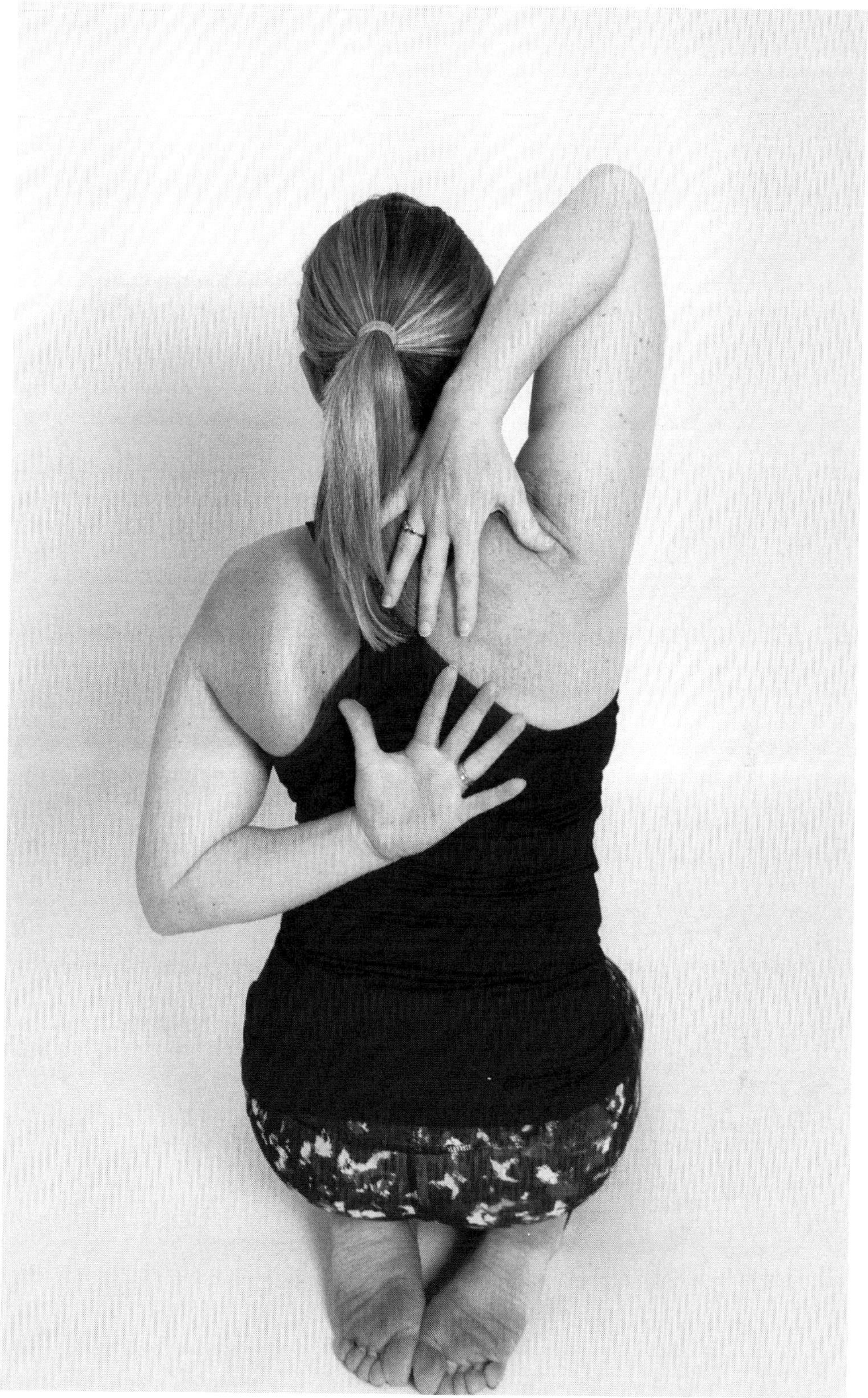

Mini Press Up on Floor

- Start on all fours, hands underneath the shoulders and knees slightly further back than the hips.

- Allow the natural curves in your spine to sit comfortably.

- **Inhale** to prepare.

- **Exhale** and bend your elbows directing the chest down in between the thumbs.

- **Inhale** to return to the start.

- **Exhale** to repeat.

- Repeat eight times.

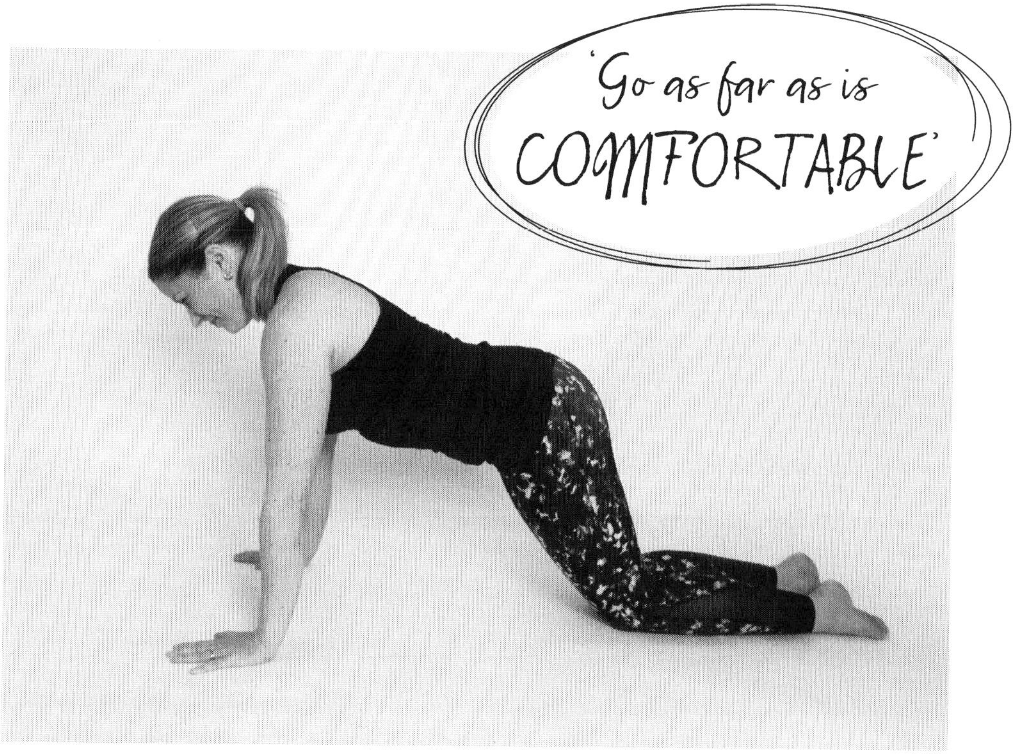
'Go as far as is
COMFORTABLE'

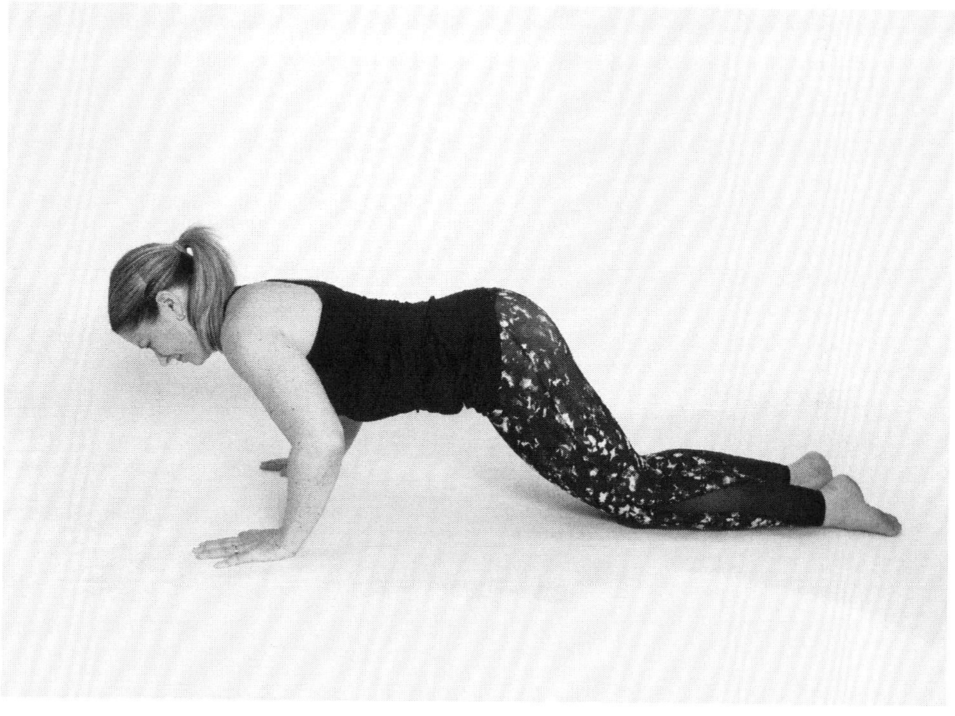

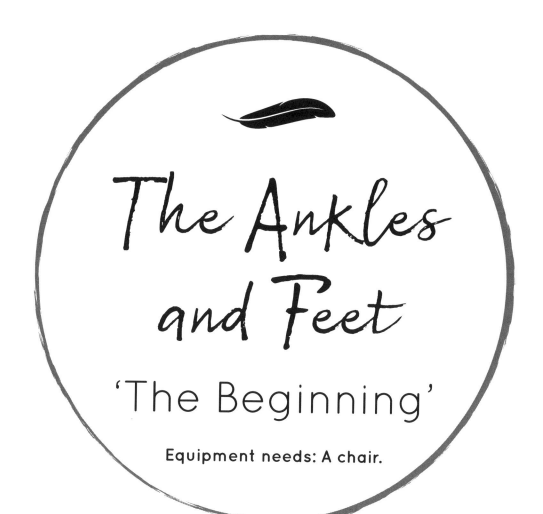

The Ankles and Feet

'The Beginning'

Equipment needs: A chair.

Ankle Turn In/ Turn Out

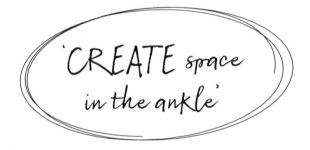

'CREATE space in the ankle'

- Stand with your hand on the back of a chair or a wall.

- Take your weight into one foot.

- **Inhale** and turn the foot out from the ankle.

- **Exhale** and turn the foot in from the ankle.

- Rest the toes on the floor if it helps.

- Repeat this eight times on each side.

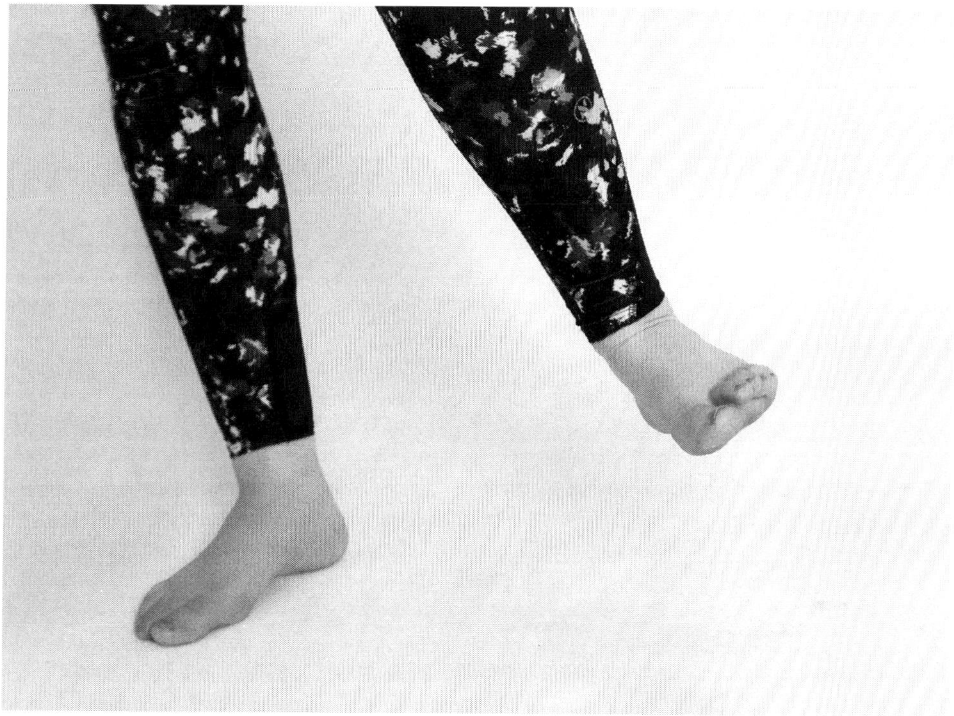

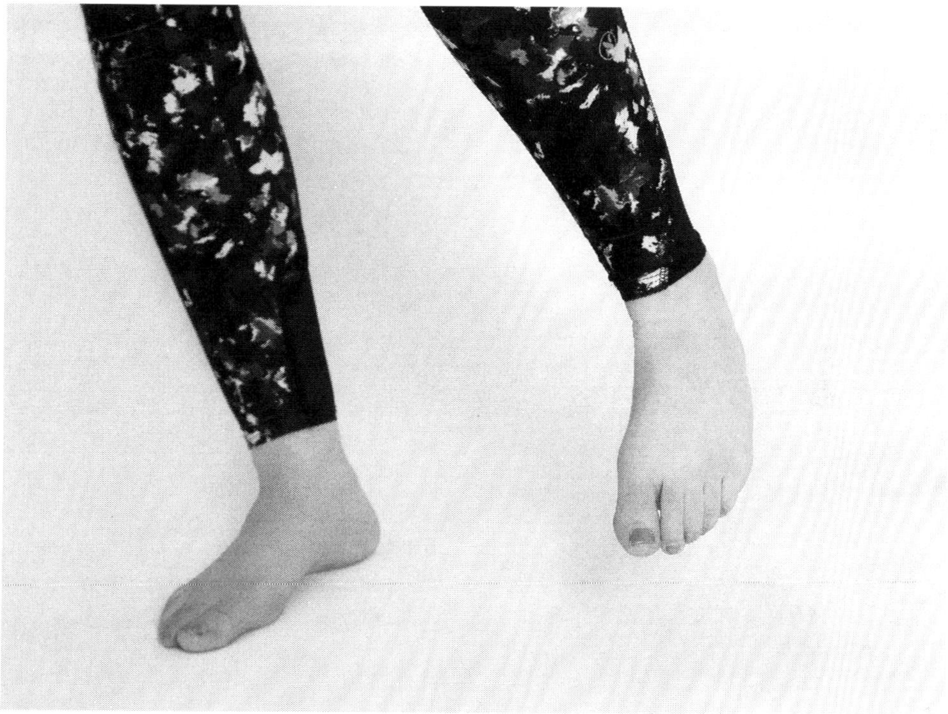

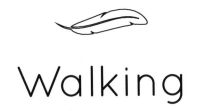

Walking

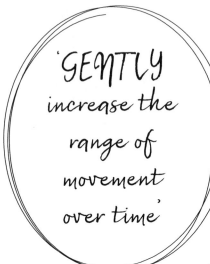

'GENTLY increase the range of movement over time'

Also useful for *'Improving'* **The Knees**

- Stand tall and balanced on both feet.

- **Inhale** and peel one heel away from the floor, stretching through the base of the toes and then lower it back down.

- **Exhale** and peel the other heel away from the floor in the same way.

- Repeat these eight times on each foot.

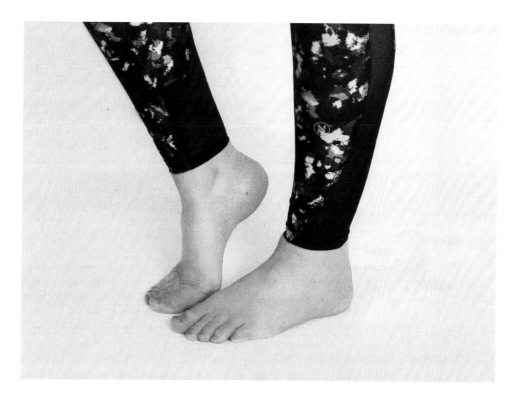

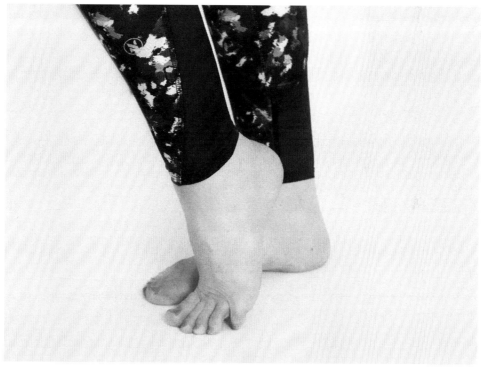

Balancing on One Foot 1

- Stand side on to the back of a chair

- Peel one heel away from the floor to a low lifted position.

- **Inhale** and **exhale** eight times as you hold this position.

- Repeat on the other side.

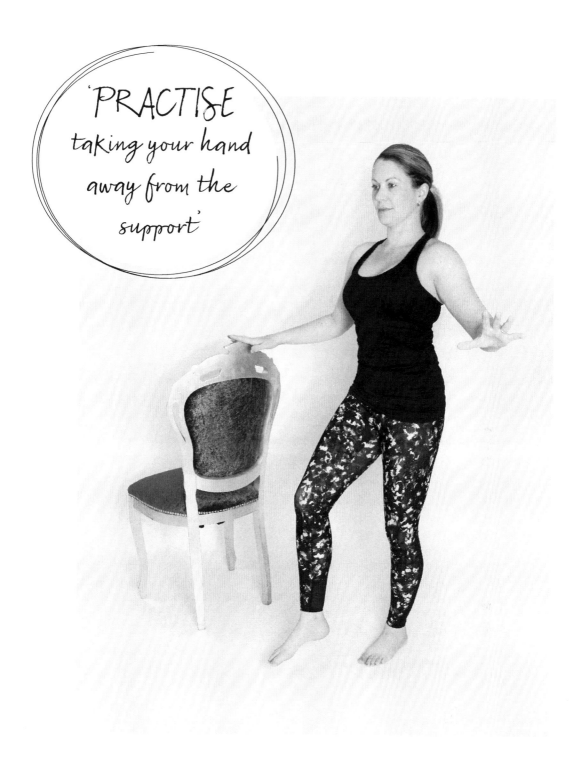

'PRACTISE taking your hand away from the support'

Scrunch and Release

- Sit with one leg out straight.

- **Inhale** as you scrunch your toes.

- **Exhale** to release.

- Repeat eight times on each side.

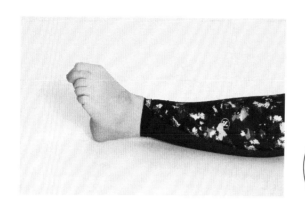

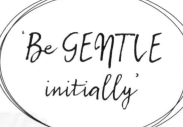

'Be GENTLE initially'

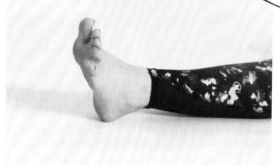

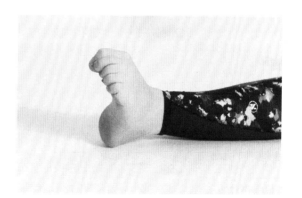

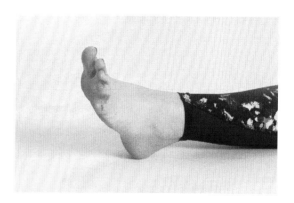

Heel Raises

- Stand tall behind the back of a chair.

- **Inhale** and peel both heels away from the floor.

- Try to come up on to the base of each big toe rather than letting the ankles roll out.

- **Exhale** to lower back down.

- Repeat eight times.

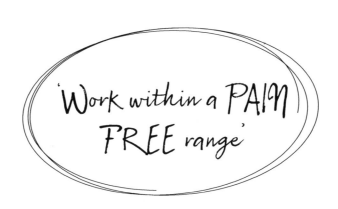

'Work within a PAIN FREE range'

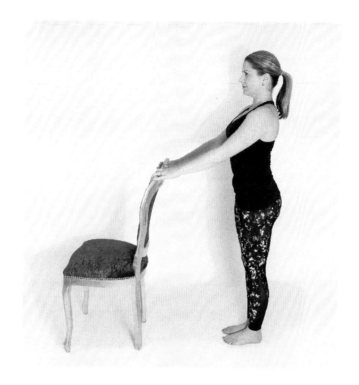

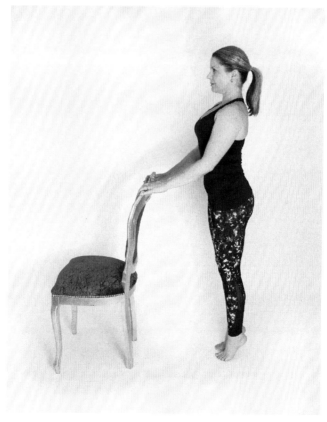

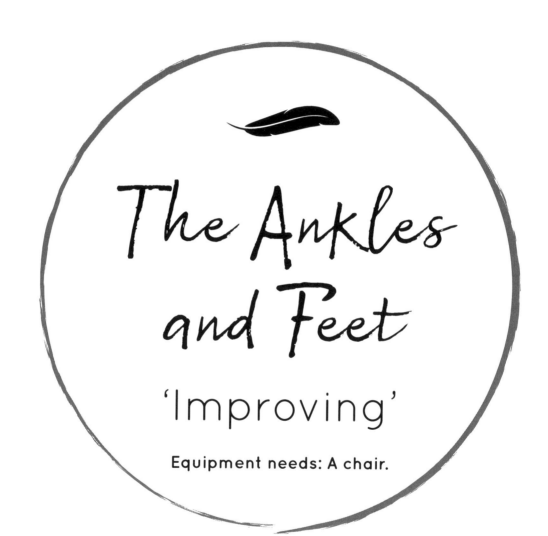

The Ankles and Feet

'Improving'

Equipment needs: A chair.

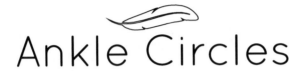

Ankle Circles

'Work within a PAIN FREE range'

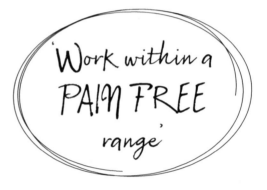

- Stand with your hand on the back of a chair or a wall.
- Take your weight into one foot.
- **Inhale** draw one full circle with the foot/ankle of the lifted foot.
- **Exhale** and draw the next circle.
- Repeat these circles eight times in each direction on both sides.

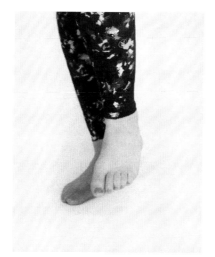 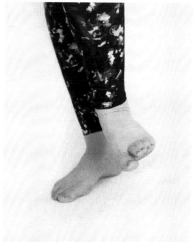

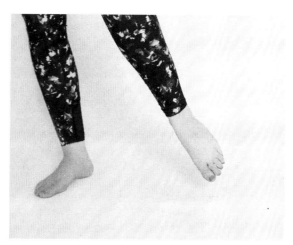

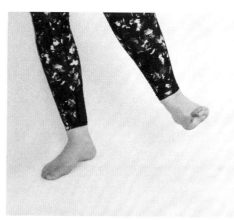 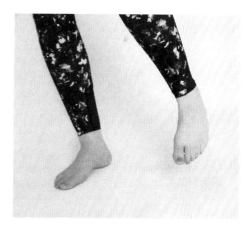

Heel Raises – parallel

- Stand tall without holding on to anything.

- Position the feet apart but in parallel.

  - **Inhale** and peel both heels away from the floor.

  - Try to come up on to the base of each big toe rather than letting the ankles roll out.

  - **Exhale** to lower back down.

  - Repeat eight times.

'IMAGINE you are leaving the crown of your head on the ceiling when you lower'

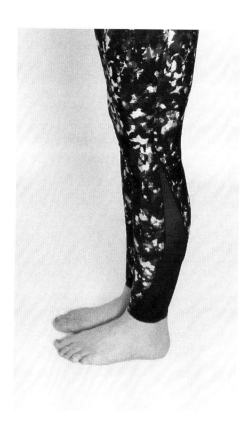
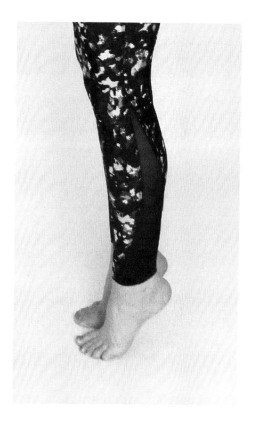

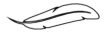

Balancing on One Foot 2

CONCENTRATE
on a spot in front of you

- Stand tall with your arms out to the side for balance.

- Peel one heel away from the floor and lift the knee up.

- **Inhale** and **exhale** eight times as you hold this position.

- Repeat on the other side.

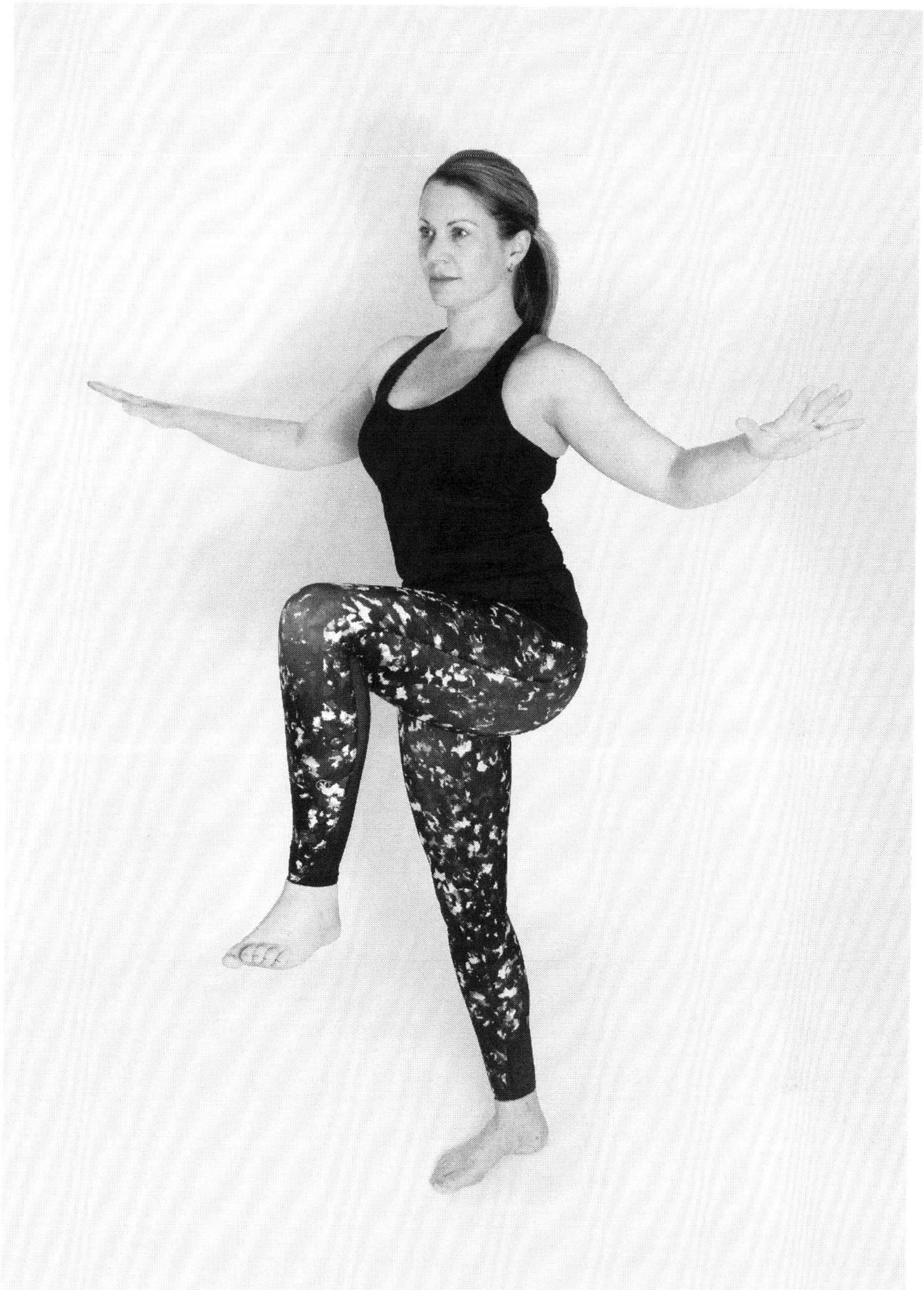

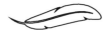

Pick up a Pen(cil)

- Place a pen or pencil on the floor.

- **Inhale** and use your toes to pick up the pen or pencil and place it down elsewhere.

- *Exhale to repeat.*

- **Repeat** eight times on each side.

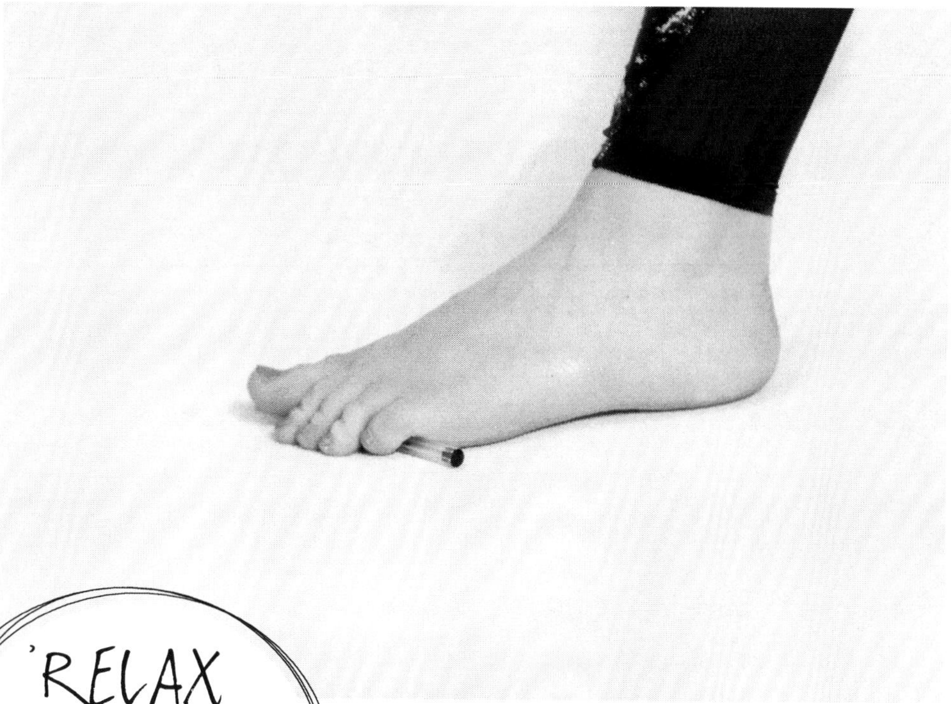

'RELAX
in the rest of
your body'

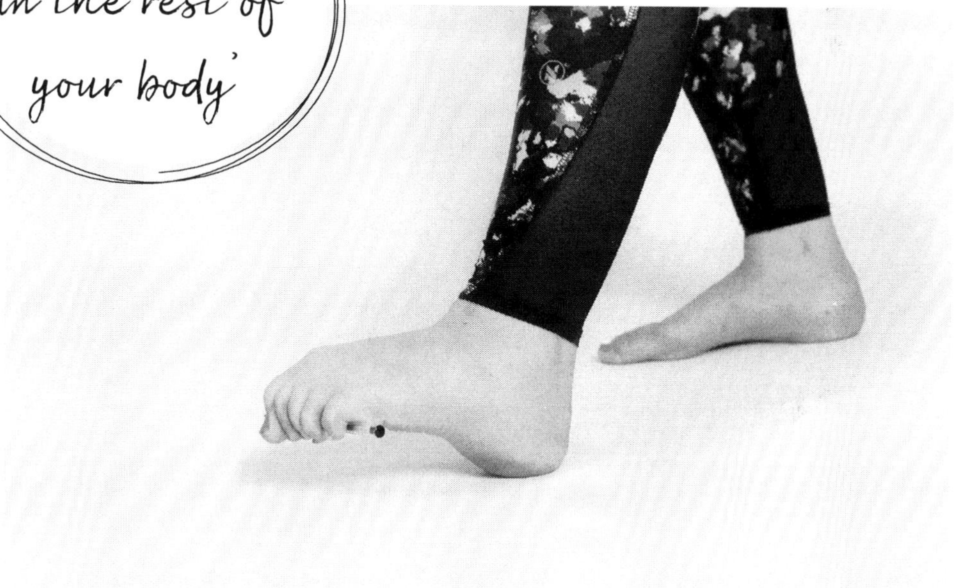

Mexican Wave for Feet

- Place your foot flat on the floor.

- **Inhale** start by lifting up your big toe.

- Then the second, third, fourth and fifth toes one by one.

- **Exhale** to place each toe down again, starting with the little toe.

- Repeat eight times on each side.

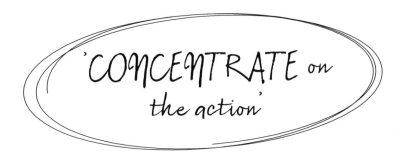

'CONCENTRATE on the action'

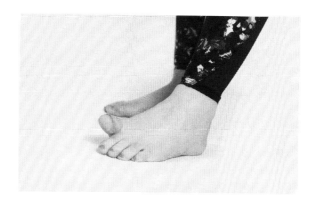

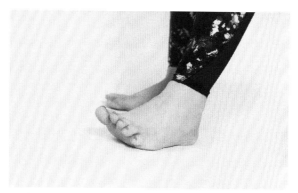

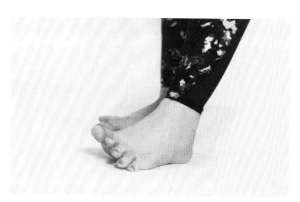

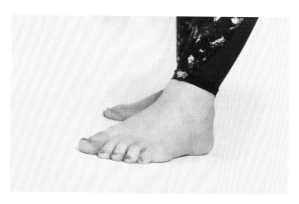

The Ankles and Feet

'Getting Better'

Equipment needs: A chair and a
bit of stretch band.

Heel Raises in Turnout

- Stand tall without holding on to anything.

- Bring your heels together and have the toes apart.

- **Inhale** and peel both heels away from the floor.

- Try to come up on to the base of each big toe rather than letting the ankles come apart.

- **Exhale** to lower back down.

- Repeat eight times.

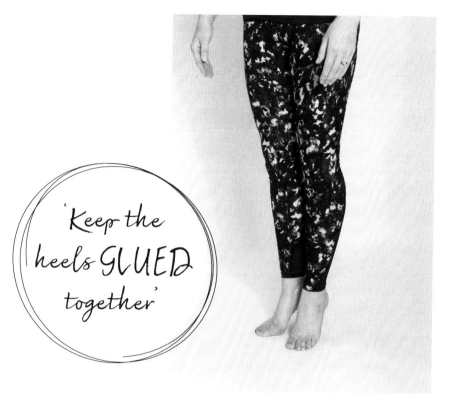

'Keep the heels GLUED together'

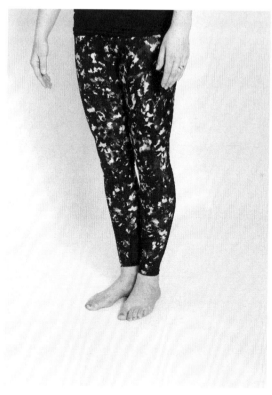

Single Leg Heel Raise

- Stand side on to the back of a chair.

- **Inhale** and peel one heel away from the floor to a high lifted position.

- **Exhale** and rise up on to the toes of the foot that is still on the floor.

- **Inhale** to lower.

- Repeat eight times on each side.

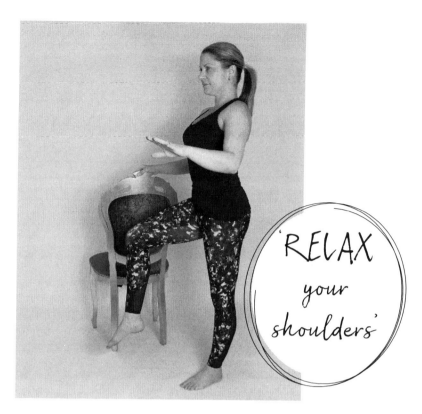

'RELAX
your
shoulders'

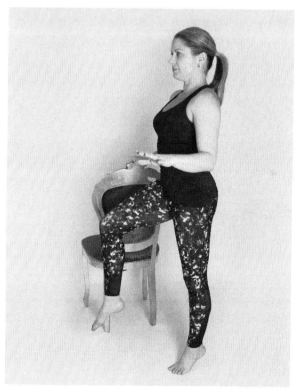

Cherry Picking

- Sit comfortably with one leg straight and the other leg bent out to the side.

- Place your foot in the band so that the toes are covered.

- **Inhale** push your foot into a point.

- *Scrunch the toes like you are 'picking cherries'.*

- **Exhale** to keep the toes scrunched and pull backwards (send the heel away).

- *Relax the toes.*

  - Repeat eight times on each side.

Optional:

  - Reverse the action.

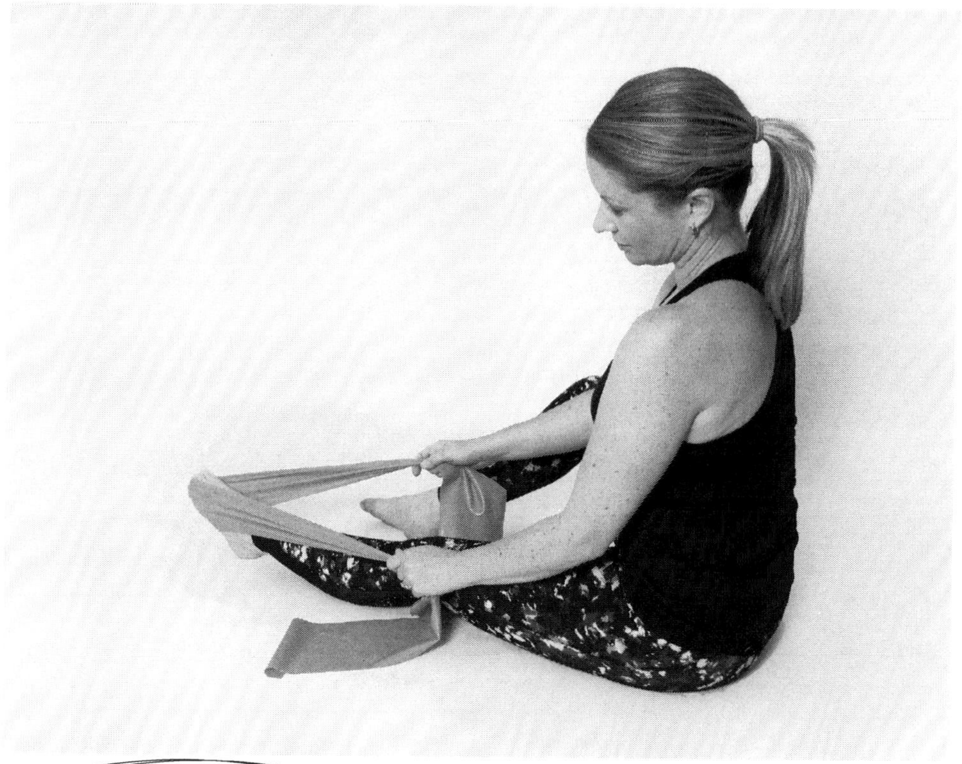

'Stay LONG through the spine'

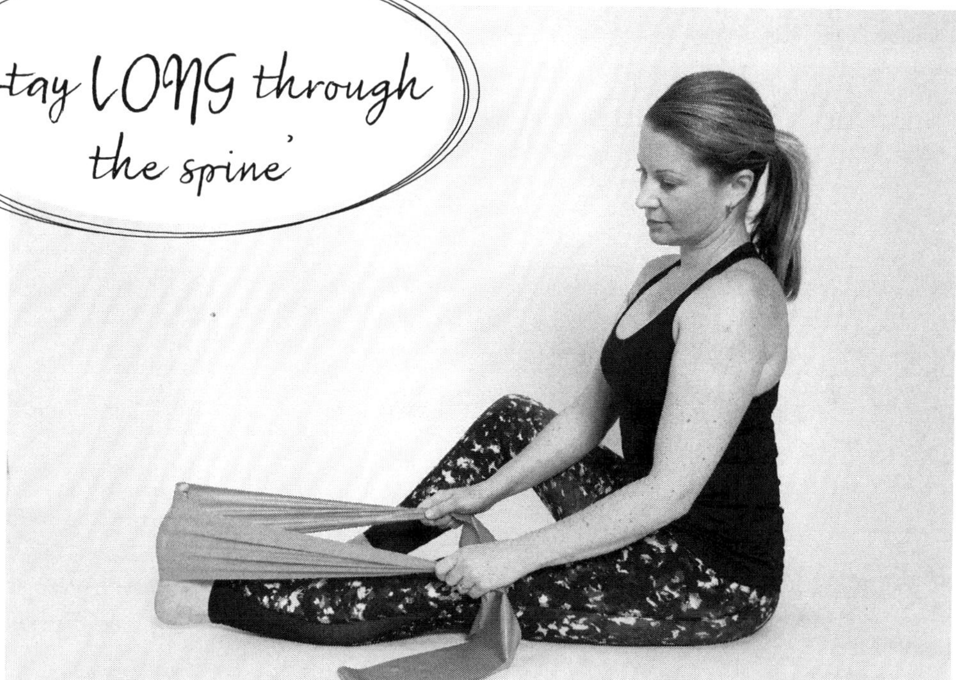

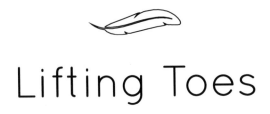

Lifting Toes

- Stand side on to the back of a chair.

- **Inhale** to prepare.

- **Exhale** to peel the toes away from the floor, standing only on the heels.

- **Inhale** to lower.

- Repeat eight times.

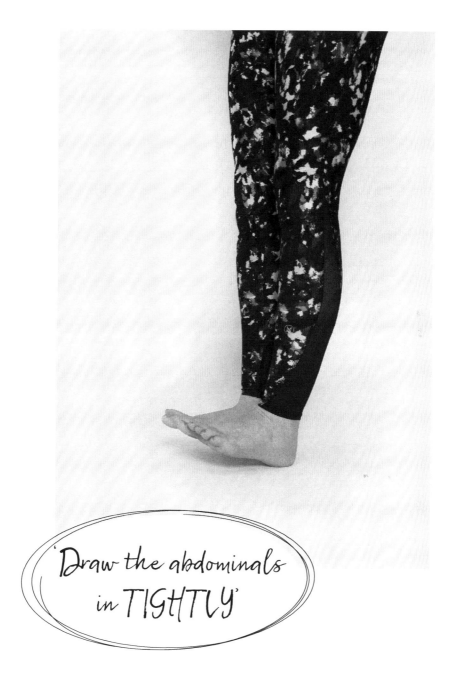

'Draw the abdominals in TIGHTLY'

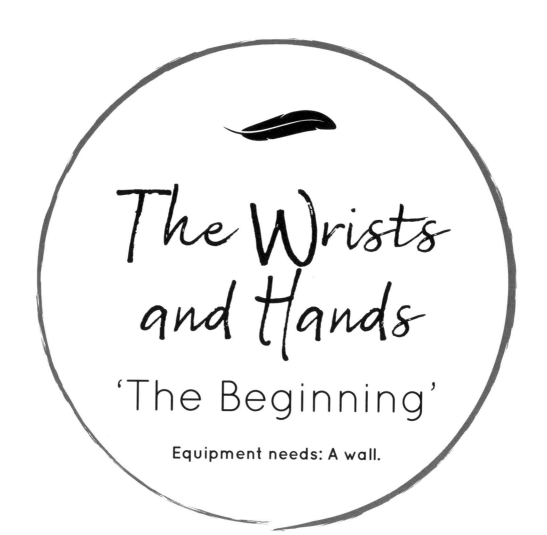

The Wrists and Hands

'The Beginning'

Equipment needs: A wall.

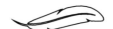

Making Fists

- Sit or stand comfortably.

  - **Inhale** to squeeze your hand into a fist.

  - **Exhale** relax the hand

  - **Inhale** to repeat.

  - Repeat eight times on each side.

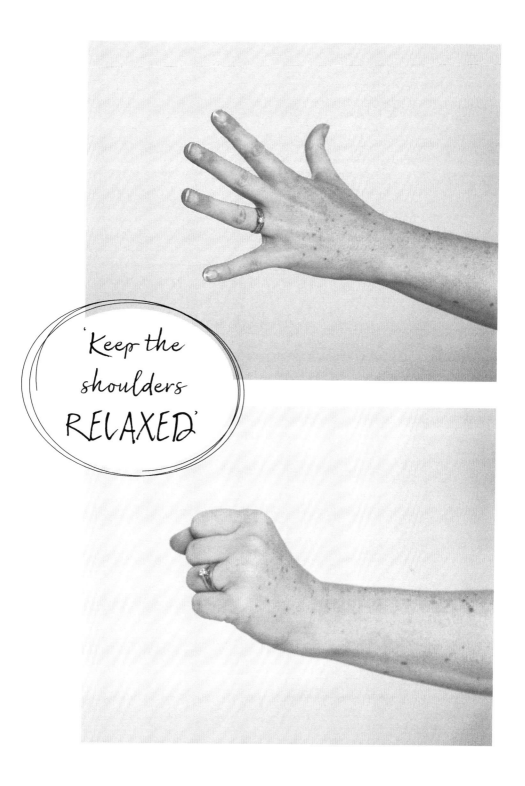

'Keep the shoulders RELAXED'

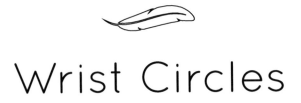

Wrist Circles

'MAINTAIN the length in the spine'

- Sit or stand comfortably.

- **Inhale** to perform one full rotation of the wrist.

- **Exhale** to circle again.

- Repeat in this way for eight circles in each direction.

- Repeat on the other side.

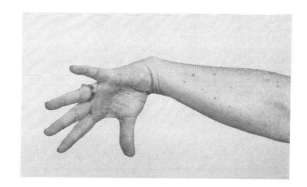

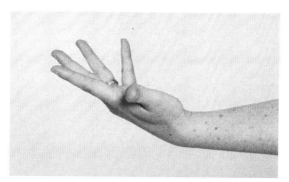

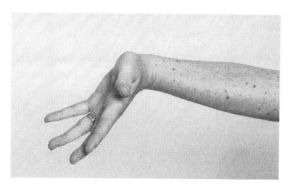

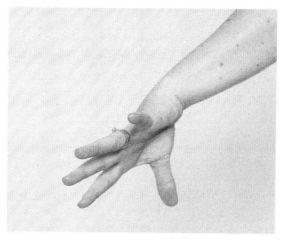

Mexican Wave for Hands

- Place your hand flat on the floor or on a surface in front of you.

- **Inhale** to lift the thumb first.

- Then the second finger, third finger, ring finger and little finger one at a time.

- **Exhale** to place the fingers back down again one at a time starting with the little finger.

- Repeat eight times on each side.

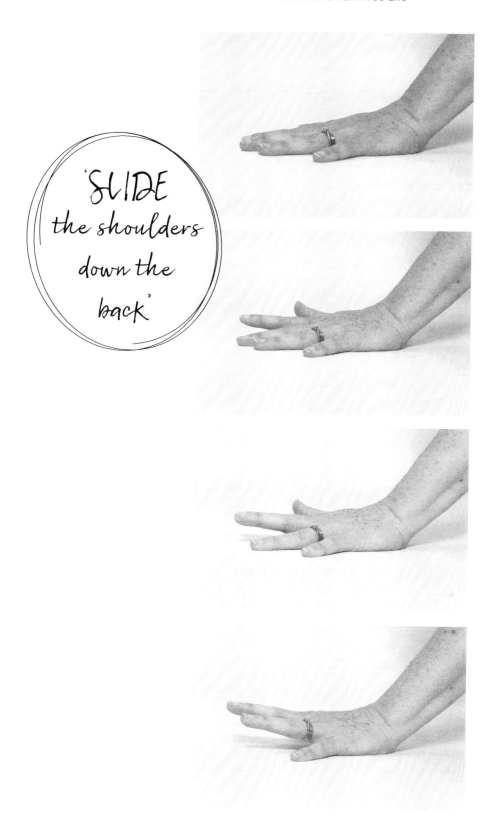

'SLIDE
the shoulders
down the
back'

Hand Against the Wall – palm flat

- Place one hand with the palm flat on the wall.

- *Lean gently into the hand, stretching through the fingers.*

- **Inhale** and **exhale** eight times as you hold the stretch.

- Repeat for eight breath rounds on the other side.

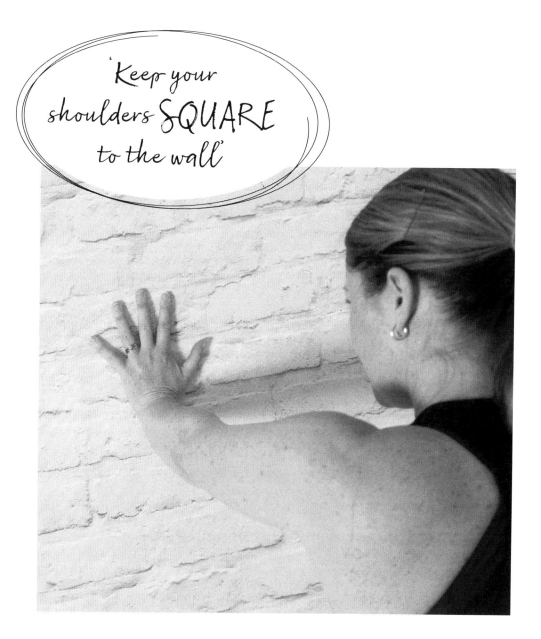

'Keep your shoulders SQUARE to the wall'

Hand Against the Wall – back of the hand

- Place one hand with the back of the hand on the wall.

- *Lean gently into the hand, stretching through the wrist and forearm.*

- **Inhale** and **exhale** eight times as you hold the stretch.

- Repeat for eight breath rounds on the other side.

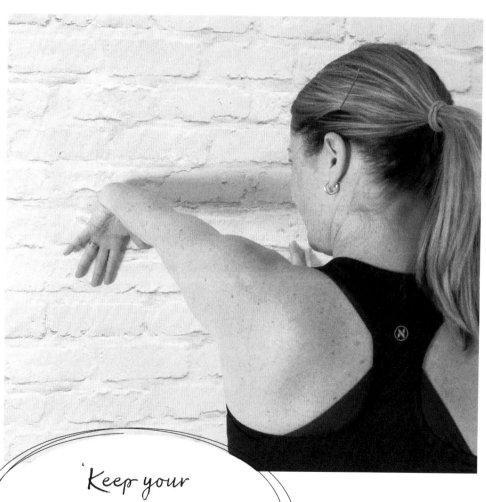

'Keep your shoulders SQUARE to the wall'

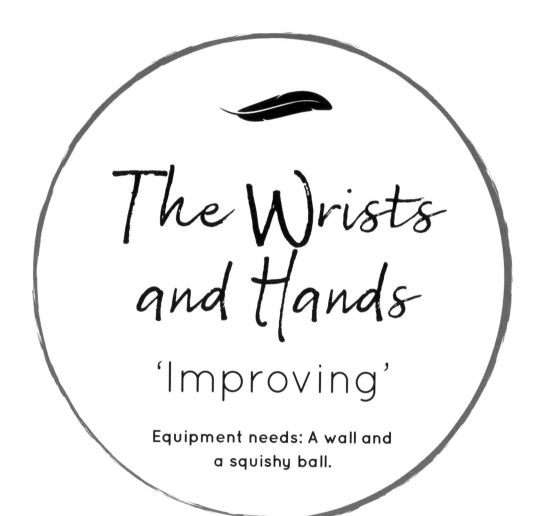

The Wrists and Hands

'Improving'

Equipment needs: A wall and a squishy ball.

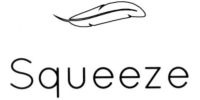

Squeeze

- Place one hand on your squishy ball.

- *Lean gently on to the ball.*

- **Inhale** and squeeze the ball tightly.

- **Exhale** to release the fingers.

- Repeat eight times on each side.

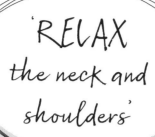

'RELAX
the neck and
shoulders'

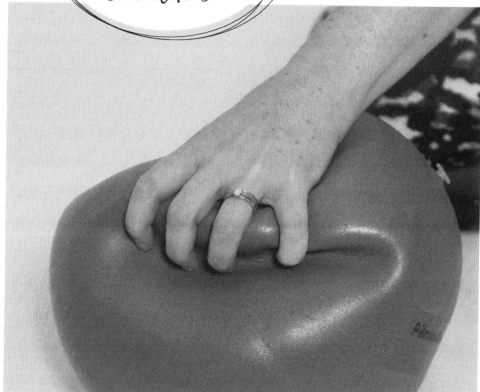

Single Hand on Floor - palm flat

- Place one hand on the floor palm flat.

- *Lean gently into the hand.*

- **Inhale** and **exhale** eight times as you hold the stretch.

- Repeat on the other side.

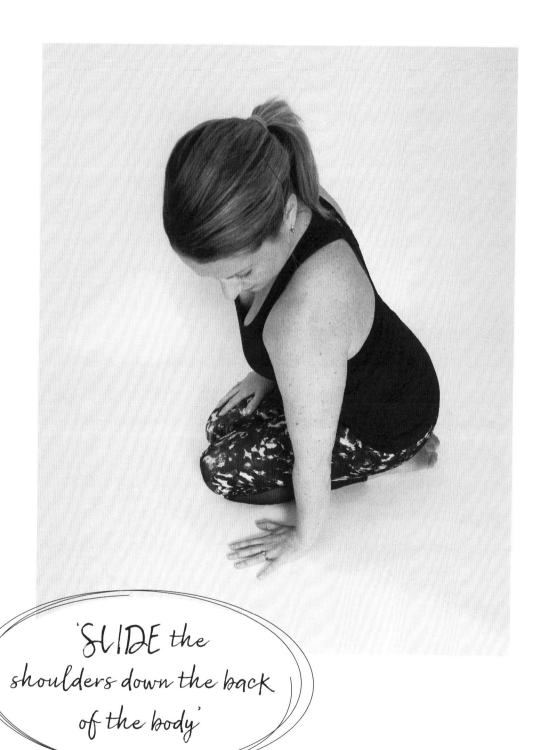

'SLIDE the shoulders down the back of the body'

Single Hand on Floor – back of the hand flat

- Place one hand on the floor, back of the hand flat.

- Lean gently into the hand.

- **Inhale** and exhale eight times as you hold the stretch.

- Repeat on the other side.

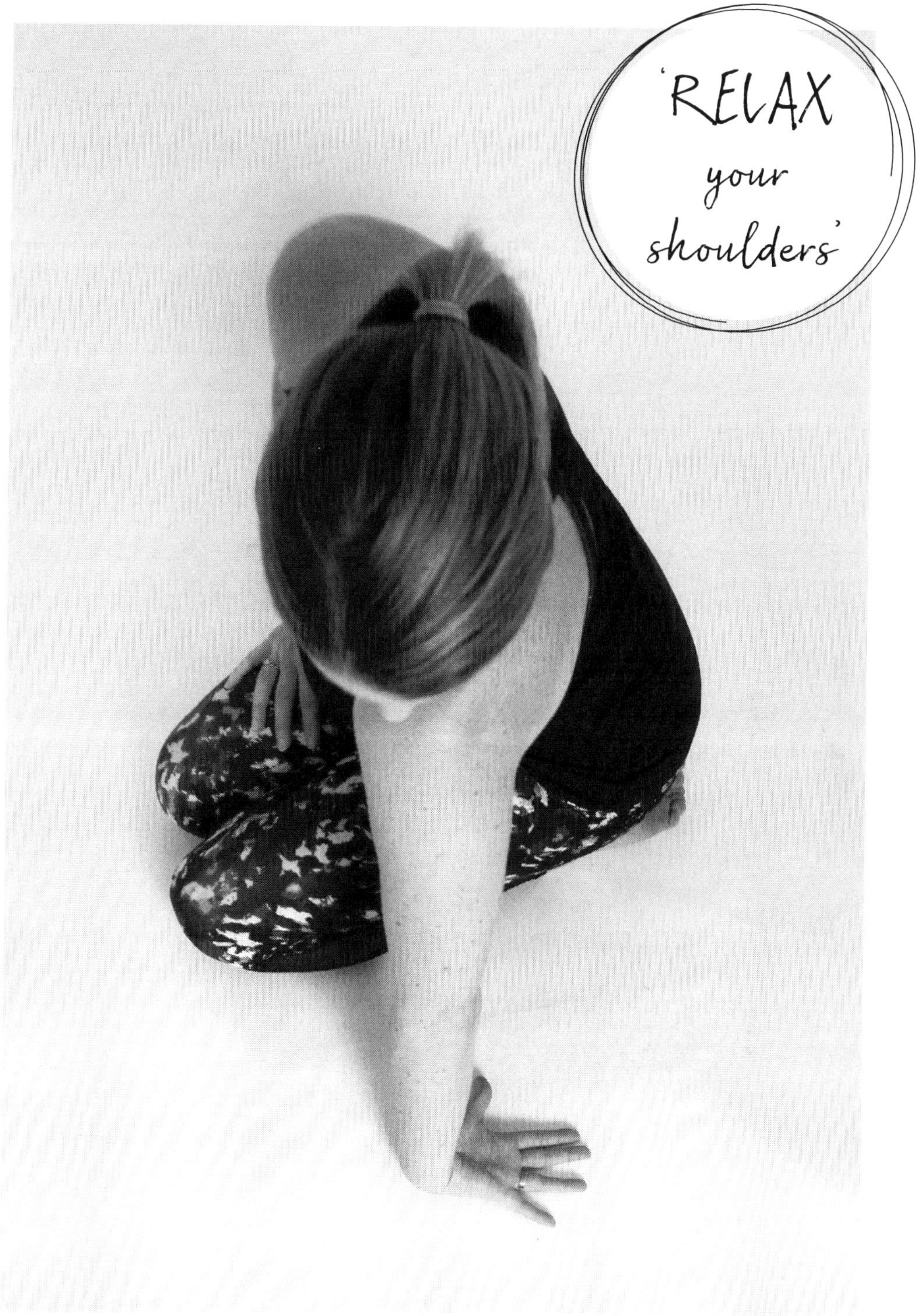
'RELAX
your
shoulders'

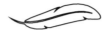

Finger Stretch

- Either sit or stand in a comfortable position.

- *Hold both arms out in front of you.*

  - Press the fingers against each other to stretch them through.

  - **Inhale** and **exhale** eight times as you hold the stretch.

'MAINTAIN
the length of
your spine'

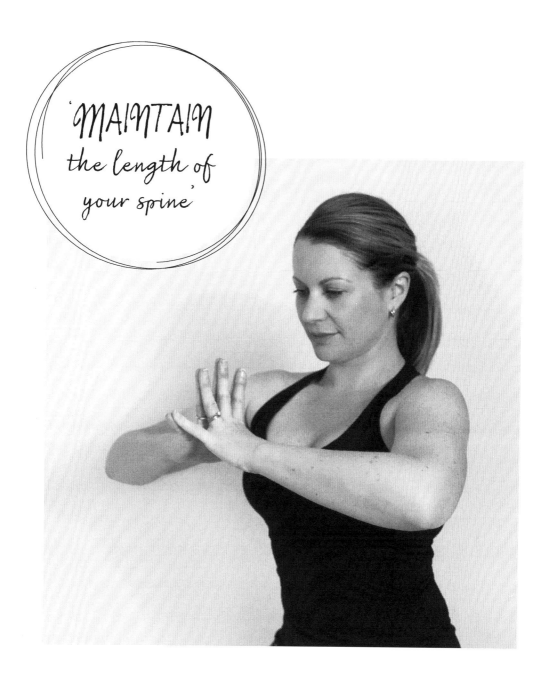

Forearm Stretch

Also useful for *'The Beginning'* **The Elbows**

- Stand facing a wall and place the back of your hand against it.

- Lean gently into the hand.

- **Inhale** and **exhale** eight times as you hold the stretch.

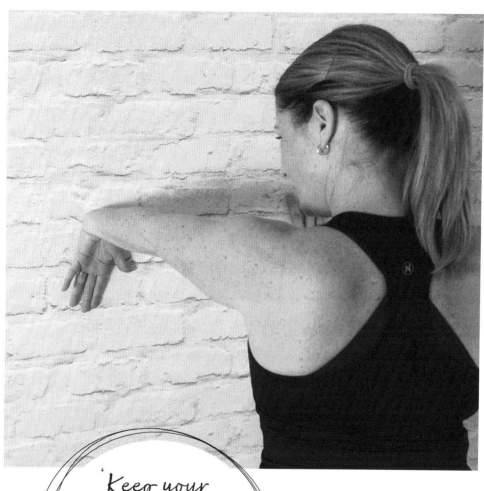

'Keep your
shoulders
SQUARE to
the wall'

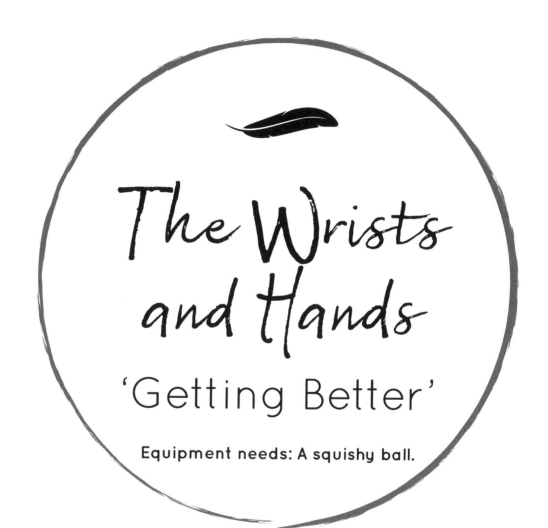

The Wrists and Hands

'Getting Better'

Equipment needs: A squishy ball.

Table Top - palms flat

- Start on all fours, palms of the hands flat and underneath the shoulders.

- Knees underneath the hips.

- Allow the natural curves in your spine to sit comfortably.

- Lean gently into the hands.

- **Inhale** and **exhale** eight times as you hold the stretch.

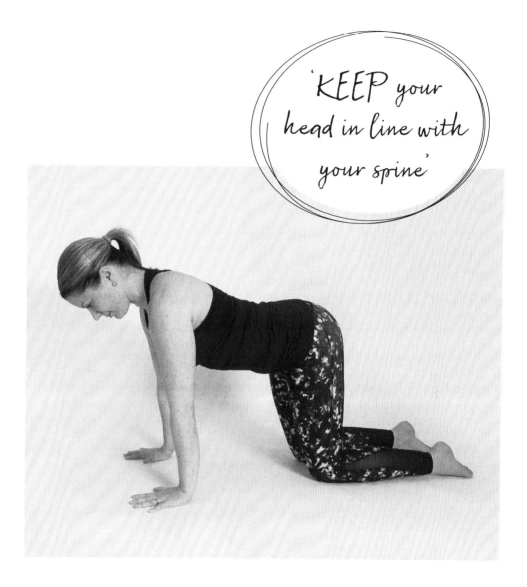

'KEEP your head in line with your spine'

Table Top – backs of hands flat

- Start on all fours, backs of the hands flat and underneath the shoulders.

- Knees underneath the hips.

- Allow the natural curves in your spine to sit comfortably.

- *Lean gently into the hands.*

  - **Inhale** and **exhale** eight times as you hold the stretch.

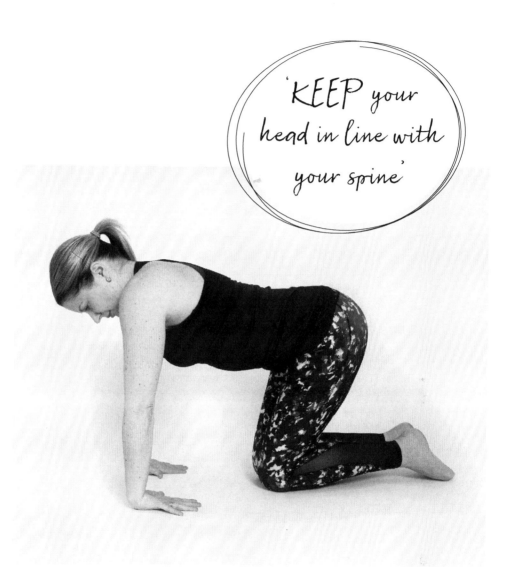

'KEEP your head in line with your spine'

Squishy Ball Press and Squeeze

- Start on all fours with one hand on the squishy ball.

- Knees underneath the hips.

- **Inhale** to lean gently into the ball and squeeze the fingers.

- **Exhale** to release the squeeze.

- Repeat eight times on each side.

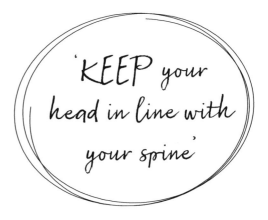

'KEEP your head in line with your spine'

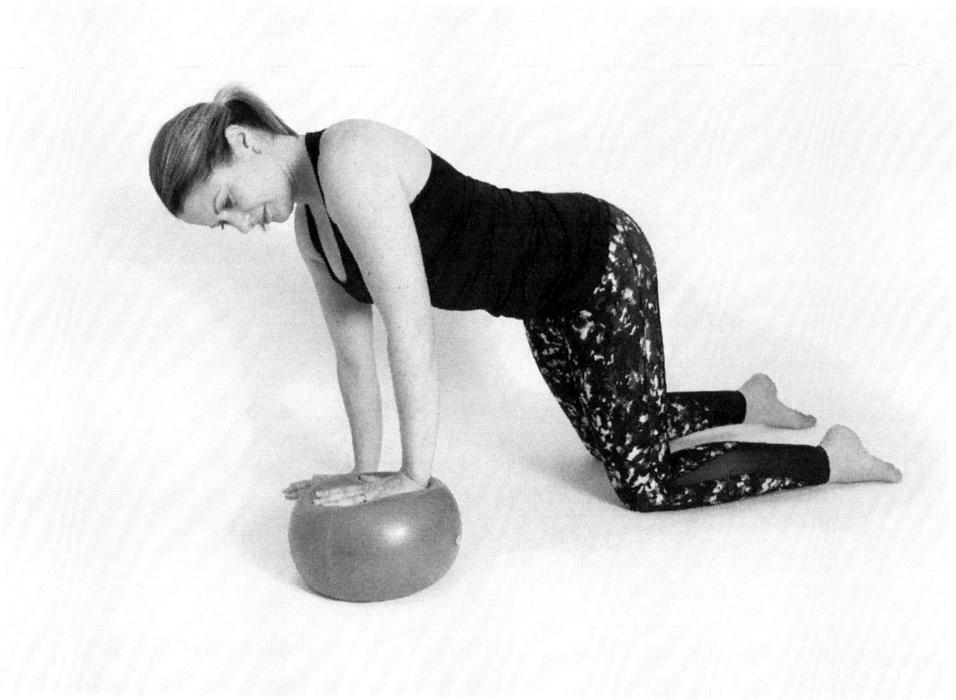

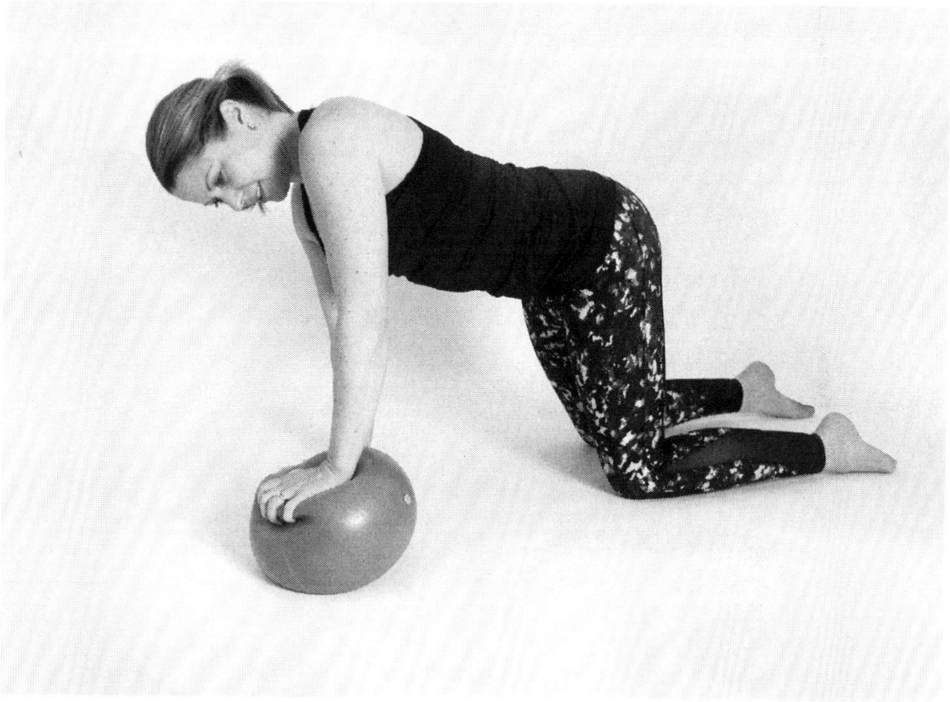

Reach Up

- Either sit or stand in a comfortable position.

- **Inhale** and lace the fingers together and push the palms away from you.

- **Exhale** and stretch both arms above the head.

- **Inhale** and **exhale** eight times as you hold the stretch.

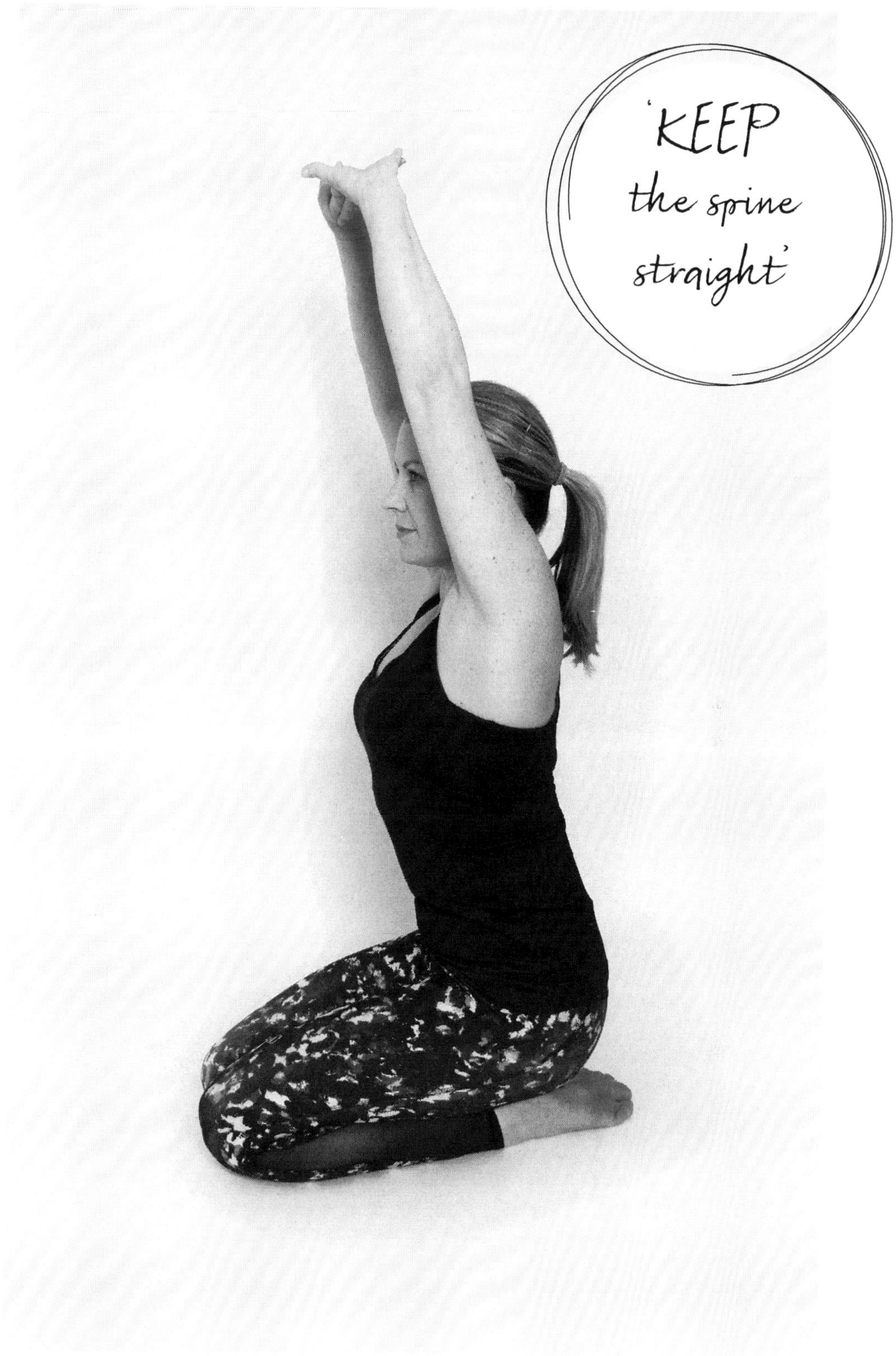
'KEEP
the spine
straight'

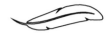

Hands Behind the Back

- Either sit or stand in a comfortable position.

- **Inhale** and take the hands behind your lower back.

- **Exhale** and try to press the palms together.

- **Inhale** and **exhale** eight times as you hold the stretch.

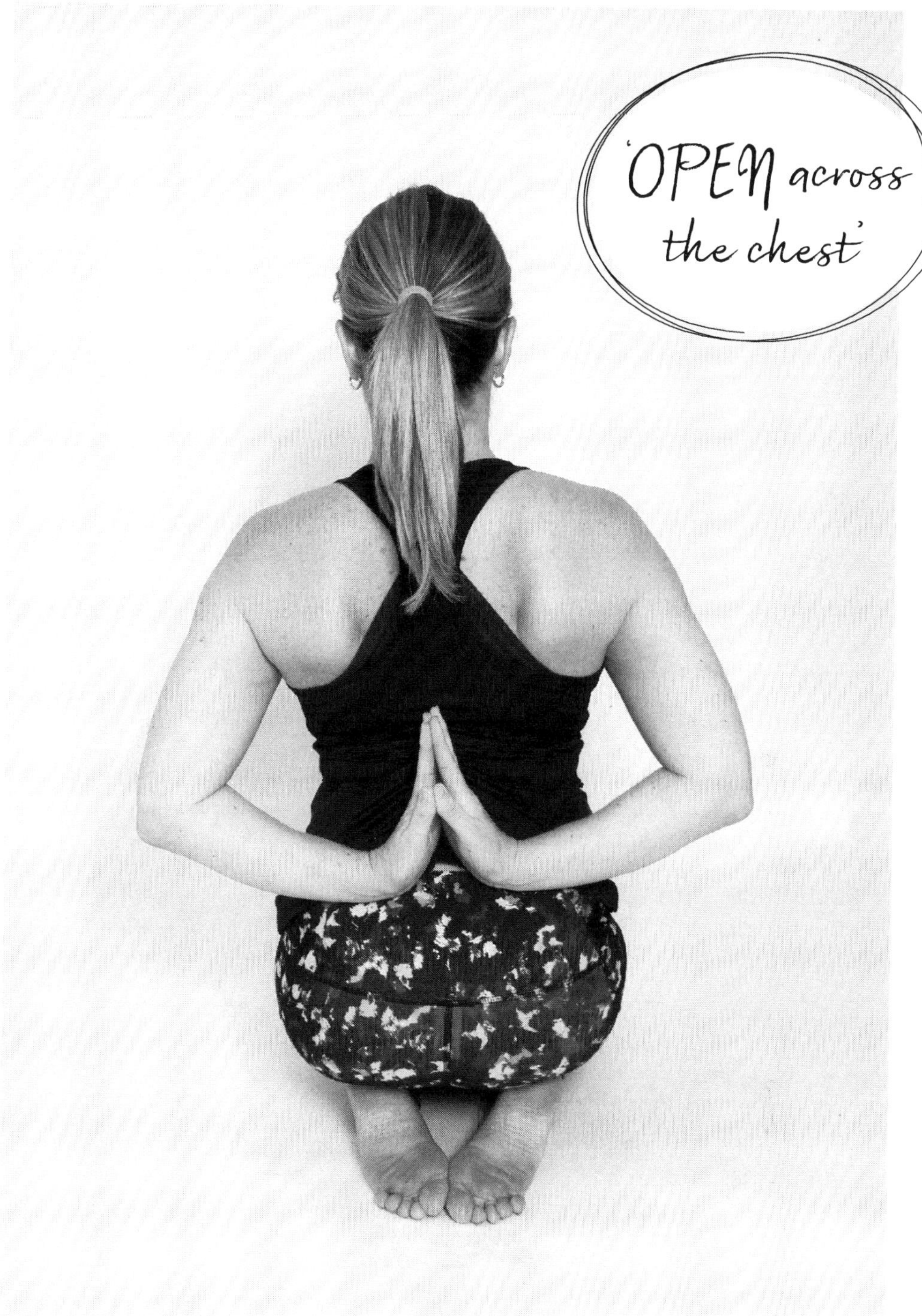
'OPEN across the chest'

About the Author

Marie-Claire Stanmore (Prettyman) lives in Southampton with her husband Mark, son Dylan and Jack Russell, Busby.

She teaches both Pilates and Yoga in groups and privately from home and from a small studio as well as training new teachers. She is also a sports massage therapist and specialises in the management of chronic pain conditions across all the disciplines.

www.themovementspecialist.co.uk

the_movement_specialist

@PilatesYogaMC

The Movement Specialist

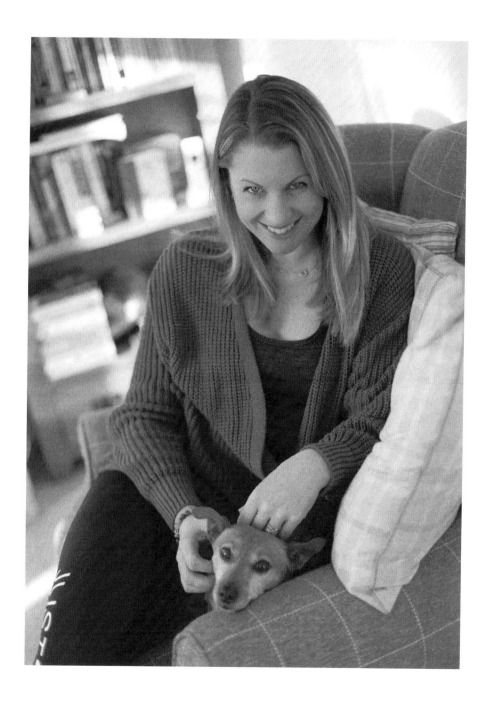